Joy and Comfort through Stretching and Relaxing

Joy and Comfort through

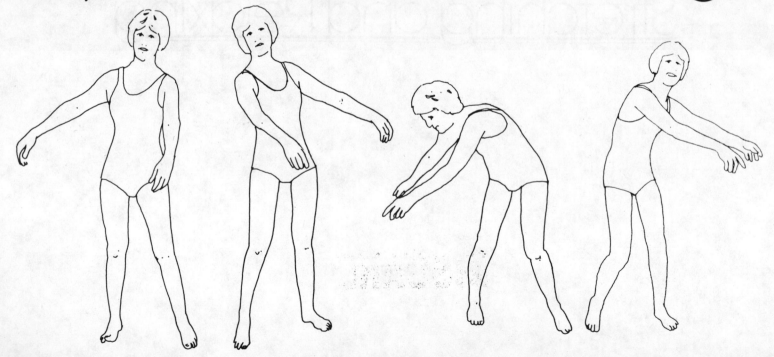

Stretching and Relaxing

FOR THOSE WHO ARE UNABLE TO EXERCISE

Ursula Hodge Casper

illustrated by Frances Boynton

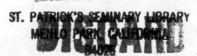

The Seabury Press / New York

To Rao

1982
The Seabury Press
815 Second Avenue
New York, N.Y. 10017
Printed in the United States of America

Library of Congress Cataloging in Publication Data
Casper, Ursula Hodge.
  Joy and comfort through stretching and relaxing.
  Includes bibliographical references.
  1. Exercise for the aged.   2. Stretch (Physiology)
3. Relaxation.   I. Title.
RA781.C33   613.7   81-18474
ISBN 0-8164-2403-9   AACR2
This book was designed by
members of the Art Department of The Seabury Press

*Grateful acknowledgment is made for the use of the following
materials:*

*Progressive Relaxation by Edmund Jacobson. Copyright ©
1938. Reprinted by permission of The University of Chicago
Press.*

Basic Human Physiology, Normal Function and Basis of
Disease. *by Dr. Arthur Guyton. Copyright © 1977. Used by
permission of W. B. Saunders Company.*

The Tao of Physics *by Fritjof Capra. Copyright © 1975. Used
by permission of Shambhala Publications, Inc.*

The Lives of a Cell *by Lewis Thomas. Copyright © 1974. Used
by permission of The Viking Press.*

"Attracting Assault: Victims Nonverbal Clues" by Betty
Grayson and Morris Stein in "The Journal of Communication," vol. 31, nbr. 1, Winter 1981. Copyright © 1981 by the
Annenberg School of Communication, University of Pennsyl-
vania, 3620 Walnut Street c-5, Philadelphia, Pa. 19104.

Drawings on pages 15, 29, and 87 by Nancy Jordan.
Drawing on page 56 by Roberta Wood.

Contents

Acknowledgments

I wish to thank all of my pupils, who, over many years, have added greatly to my understanding and knowledge. Without pupils, how can any teacher learn?

William Potier, insisting that others who teach classes in movement would be interested in my ideas, initiated the thought of this book and urged me to continue writing it.

A debt of gratitude is also due to Emeritus College of the College of Marin, California, for starting the class "Autobiography, Writing from Experience," and to Eugenie Yaryan, the instructor, for saying to me, "Of course you can write."

Josephine Carson, my teacher for the last three years, labored valiantly to teach me the art of writing, and to her my gratitude is boundless.

My friend and colleague, Mary Sue Fitzgerald, warrants enormous appreciation for her constant encouragement and her editorial and typing skills.

❧ CHAPTER ONE ❧

Waking Up
to Body Awareness

I hope that this book brings you recipes for comforting your body when you feel stiff, have pains here and there, or when you just don't want to move. There are periods for all of us when life seems very dusty when we are discouraged.

This is a scary time in which to live. We recoil from the world of violence all around us. We do not want to be identified with the world of hate. We need to love, love deeply, with positive feelings about ourselves and about others, with feelings of strength rather than despair.

Probably, it was my own need to develop feelings of strength that led me, these forty years, first to teach and then to write about the movements and ideas that you will find here. The hope that this book will strengthen your self esteem, thus your ability to give love to others, is my gift to you.

I want to tell you the personal story of my life, because I cannot convey in any other way the depth of my feelings about the importance of being truly aware of our bodies, of movement, and of conscious relaxation.

In the mid-1930s I became totally exhausted and developed an ugly, magenta-colored butterfly rash on my face. I was told I had Lupus Erythematosus, then a little-understood disease that was thought to be incurable, with a life expectancy of from two to fourteen years. Today, it is known that Lupus is an auto-immune disease, in which the victim generates anti-bodies that attack his own cells. You might say that the victim destroys himself. New drugs have been found to control the disease, and life expectancy has lengthened. Obviously, this illness influenced my life tremendously.

I was pregnant when the disease was diagnosed. It was a relief to know that there *was* reason for me to feel so badly, that I was not "just rejecting my pregnancy" as some friends insisted. Because I felt too tired to read, I spent my time in bed, finding and relaxing the muscles of my body.

I remember, at first, I spent a lot of time with my toes, stretching them, trying to move one toe at a time, and finally letting them become loose. Then I discovered that I could tighten and loosen the muscles of the calves of my legs and then the muscles near my shin bones. I had been a dancer, so had some knowledge of muscles, but never before had I had the leisure to investigate them.

The muscles of my lower back were particularly fascinating: I found that if I could loosen the muscles extending from the last lumbar vertebra down to and including the muscles surrounding the anus, I experienced a great sense of relief. When I could maintain this looseness long enough, I would fall asleep. Even today I still find this hard to think about while remaining alert enough to write.

My baby was born very quickly and easily. The doctor wasn't there, because he had said that I would have a long hard labor. I had gone to the hospital early, because I had had a dream that said I should. In 1944 I read the first book on pregnancy written for the layman that I had ever seen. In it I learned that my delivery had been easy because my pelvic muscles were so relaxed that they did not impede the emergence of the baby.

After World War II, I was hired by two obstetricians in San Francisco who were pioneering the idea of training women for childbirth. I was allowed neither to teach movement nor talk about labor. I did not have a degree. However, I was permitted to teach muscular relaxation to their patients. This was the beginning of a great learning experience, and I am grateful to these doctors.

After a few years I became ill again and retired to Marin County. When I felt better, I began teaching classes in my home or in any place I could find to prepare women for childbirth. Now I was free, not only to teach movement, but to discuss labor as well as muscular relaxation. It was during these early days that I worked out movements that would help women discover, and loosen, that vital low back area.

Years later I found that these movements were helpful to older women as well as to younger. I speak of older women because older men tend not to join classes in body awareness. I found that in a class of thirty, two men would join twenty-eight women. Some men had lots of courage: I remember one retired professor, stiff and tense, who after a few semesters working with me went on to join a class in modern dance.

During my thirty years of teaching, I found that the barrier, sometimes insurmountable, against moving and relaxing was a cultural one, inherited, in our country, I suppose, from our Puritan fathers. "How abominable and filthy is man," the Bible says. Cotton Mather, a famous New England preacher, wrote in his diary in his fiftieth year, 1712, "Excretory Necessities of Nature should be still accompanied with some holy thought of a Repenting and abased Soul." This feeling about the body still persists.

Recently I was asked to talk about exercise and relaxation to a small senior group meeting in a church basement. We sat in a circle, and an old man sitting next to me began muttering. At first I didn't quite understand what he was saying, something about "the house of God." I was describing ways of moving to help stretch painful spots when he said, loudly, "You're talking vile." I asked why and he answered, "That's evil talk."

I suppose speaking of the body implies sexual intercourse to many, but to me, body awareness means awareness of every waking minute, to experience walking, running, sitting down and standing up, breathing, stretching, bending. It means feeling pain as well as pleasure and laughter. It means recognizing the feeling of fatigue, as well as the bliss of rest when the body asks for it. It means knowing that the body is *us* in this dimension that we call reality.

When I was young I was told, "Don't think about yourself. Think about others. If you think about others you won't have time to think about yourself." This part of my social training was designed to combat shyness, but the meaning I perceived was, "I'm not worth thinking about. Everyone else is worthy." I know I was not alone in this perception, since many of my pupils have said: "Oh, but it's not *nice* to think about yourself."

"Love your neighbor as yourself" is a beautiful rule. I have no quarrel with it except that it was always translated, to me at least, as "Love your neighbor, but do *not* love yourself." It took me years to learn that it really means, "Love your neighbor *and* yourself. Love completely, with no judgments, no reservations, no resentment. When you love yourself you have more love to give to your neighbor." Loving your body means caring for it, attending to it, treating it as a good friend.

If we don't love our bodies, we cannot pay attention to them. Our bodies then become like small children who want to tell their mothers something, but can't because mother is busy talking to someone else. Eventually the child becomes so frustrated that she cries and mother is obliged to listen. I think our bodies do this to us. First there is a low murmur; in body language, this is a feeling of slight discomfort which we, being well conditioned to the demands of this world, brush aside and get on with our work. Later the discomfort may become a slight pain, so we take an aspirin and get on with our work. If we ignore the language of the body long enough, it may start to cry, really cry, and then we have to see a doctor who may put us in the hospital. I believe that we should treat the body as a beloved child and pay attention to what it is saying. What the slight murmur means, to me at least, is that my body is tired and wants to lie down. When I am too busy or inattentive, it devises ingenious ways to lay me low so that it can rest.

I did not, and do not, teach relaxation in the same way as Dr. Edmund Jacobson.[1] An eminent physiologist, Jacobson trained patients to contract the muscles of one arm as tightly as possible and then to let go, in order to feel those muscles relax while he followed their progress on his kymograph. I have found that stretching is a more natural way to prepare a muscle to relax, and thus have gathered and devised the following stretches. After all, we know that a cat indulges in delicious stretches before settling into an inert body.

A muscle can carry an emotional charge, or tension, held over from past fears or angers. When we are angry we become tense. We clench our fists, our arms and shoulders get ready to swat, the lower back and thighs assume the posture of a fighter, we make ourselves heavy by stiffening the whole torso. If we really had a fight—if our anger resulted in a life or death struggle—all this muscular tightening would be useful. In the fight itself we would expend our energy and stretch the clenched muscles. But physical combat no longer is the acceptable way of dealing with differences. Instead, we have verbal combats, and after one of these we are left with a stiff, tense, and uncomfortable body.

We frequently become annoyed by all the thousands of irritations besetting us in this noisy mechanical world. Without our realizing it our muscles are subtly tightening with no way to relieve the tension. It takes a muscle many times longer to relax than to tighten, and unless there is movement that will stretch the tight muscle, the tension remains as residue.

Shortly before the end of my first marriage, every evening after dinner, while I was washing the dishes, I developed hives. I had read somewhere that hives could be caused by suppressed rage. Due to my upbringing, I could not admit the rage nor identify the anger, although every time I started to itch I took the plate I was washing and dashed it into the sink, breaking it to bits. Extraordinary though it be, as I decimated the lovely set of blue and white English china, my hives lessened. When there was no more china, I had no more hives. I wish I had known then that stretching, kicking, punching pillows, and shouting would have done just as well, for I liked that china.

Later, Lama Tarthang Tulku[2] Rinpoche, founder of the Nyingma Centers in Berkeley, taught me the following technique to rid myself of anger:

Clench your hands into fists, bend your elbows and bring your fists to your chest. Now take three deep breaths and with each breath think of something that has made you angry. Breathe in, one, begin to get angry; breathe in, two, and get still more angry; breathe in, three, your rage is boundless; so throw your hands and arms apart and yell "BAH" as loudly as possible. It's a great relief!

In 1979 at a conference on "Visualization: New Dimensions in Body/Mind," conducted by the University of California Extension Division at Santa Cruz, Dr. Winifred Lucas[3] spoke of "Imagery as the Organization of Body/Mind Energy Fields." In her presentation she referred to anger as the "single hardest thing in our culture to deal with." The following is her suggestion of a way to deal with anger at a person:

> Visualize the person who is the subject of your anger and irritation. Make a mental list of those irritations. Then say to your vision of the person, "I am cancelling out these things. I know that you cannot change so I am cancelling out my expectations and accepting you as you are."

This takes practice and is not easy.

Of course, the most pervasive, negative emotion is fear. I have an intuitive notion that joy, delight in living, and its opposite, fear of living, are indigenous to all life forms. I envision protozoa moving happily toward food and then, when afraid of approaching enemies, contracting in self defense. A protozoan's life must be a constant exchange between these two extremes; to eat and to avoid being eaten are the thrusts of its life.

Analogies between protozoa and human beings are ridiculous. Of course, they cannot be compared. Yet, we are a composite of cells of living matter whose ancestors are older than we can imagine. There is a similarity; joy and fear are our life heritage.

I think the important thing about fear is that it is paralyzing. The cortex does not work well when one is afraid. "Frozen with fear" is a good description, and when one is frozen, one is tense. Fear hits the involuntary as well as the voluntary muscles. Sometimes it's insidious, because we don't recognize it. The only way to handle fear, that I know of, is to face it. Face what we are afraid of, right now, this second.

During the time when I was ill, I had an experience which illustrates this. I had moved to the country where someone had offered me a little house on a hill. In some ways I had begun to feel rested and stronger, but developed some new symptoms. I supposed that these were a new phase of my illness. However, after a few weeks I noticed that they surfaced only after I had returned to the house from shopping. At first I thought that I had become too tired when I went out, but then realized that even when I felt perfectly fine, and only drove down to the village and back, by the time I arrived home I had stomach cramps and diarrhea.

My house was reached by a narrow curving road. One day as I was driving up the hill I got such a sharp cramp in my stomach that I pulled over to a wide spot in the road and turned off the motor. I sat in the car and felt the pain, thought about the pain, went into it, then realized that the pain was fear. I was terrified—terrified of that road. I remembered then that the first time I went up that road I thought that it was pretty scary—but had put the thought out of my mind, as being unsuitable for a mother with a child. I did not want my daughter to sense the fear, so I had pushed it down below the surface of consciousness.

I realized that one of the things I feared was that the motor would die on the way up. But now the motor was off and I could walk home, if I wanted to. There was no danger. The pain began to subside. As I thought about my fear and began to understand it, it left. It was impossible to hold on to it because there was indeed nothing to fear. The fear left and the pain left. I started the motor and drove home. The pain and the diarrhea vanished.

One could say, "But what you felt wasn't really fear, it was anxiety, or worry." My dictionary says the word "worry" derives from "ME (Middle English) *worowen, wirien,* to strangle." The word, "anxious," comes from "Latin, *anxious;* Fr. *angere,* to cause pain, to choke." To be strangled or choked seems to me to be a fearsome experience. The tensions which fear, worry, anxiety and anger produce are endless and often we don't even know we have them.

The sensation of fear produces muscular tension, which greatly exacerbates pain. Physiologists and neurophysicians tell us that pain travels on certain nerves and is received at certain spots in the brain. It follows that tension (muscle tightness) adds to the pain through additional muscle contraction around the nerves. A body sensation from a traumatized part is not necessarily painful, but when the muscles surrounding that part are tightened, the sensation usually becomes painful. Often, pregnant women in the classes I taught said that when they were completely relaxed during labor, the contractions were strong and could be felt, but were not necessarily painful. When the muscles were tightened, however, it hurt like hell!

Many years ago I had a dramatic demonstration of the relation of tension to pain. I had not been feeling well and awoke one moring with a pain in my left eye. I dragged myself to an ophthalmologist who found that I had an ulcer on the cornea of my eye (i.e., a sore on my eyeball). He said I must lie quietly in bed for at least two weeks, in a room where there was no dust, smoke, cats or dogs. I must have certain drops in my eyes every hour, but the drops must be kept in the refrigerator between times. And finally he said that if I did not carry out his instructions, I would probably lose the sight of that eye and that it might spread to the other eye, a statement which I translated into the specter of total and immediate blindness.

I was terrified. I lived with my dog and three cats in a room heated by a fireplace. I called my internist and pleaded for help, but by the time I reached the hospital I was hysterical and the pain had reached unbearable intensity. A friend tried to calm me, to help me relax, but I was completely out of control and got no relief until a blessed shot knocked me out. The ulcer was slow in healing. I was hospitalized for over two weeks.

The following spring I ignored some warning signs my body had been giving me. Again, one morning I awakened with the pain in my left eye. I wasn't frightened because I knew I would be taken care of, my doctor knew what to do, the hospital was alerted that I was coming and I was given a shot before I was out of control. I stayed ten days that time, and the visit might have been shortened had I not had so much medication.

The third time I stayed in the hospital only one week and needed less medication, because I remained loose and relaxed and therefore healed quickly.

Then, there was a fourth time. I was married and happy, but, as usual doing a little more than my strength allowed. I awoke one morning with the sharp stabbing pain in my left eye. I spoke to the ophthalmologist's secretary, insisting that this was an emergency. She said that he was completely booked for three weeks and would not be in his office until one o'clock that day. I stayed in bed for awhile, then dressed very slowly and my husband drove me down at one.

The secretary was still unfriendly and wanted me to leave, but I said that I would sit in the waiting room until he could see me. She shrugged, so I sat, with my eyes not closed but unfocused (a state George Leonard[4] would later call "soft eyes"). When people in the waiting room asked about my trouble, I was able to reply honestly that I was in no pain as long as my eyes were loose.

Four and a half hours later, at five-thirty, the doctor appeared. He was furious with his staff for not telling him I was there. Anesthetic drops in my eye revealed that indeed there was an ulcer, but—the doctor found this very strange—there were indications that it had been quite a bit larger. He could hardly believe it, but the eye was healing already. After three days of my husband's loving care, the ulcer was gone, with no medication at all.

Psychoanalysts and psychiatrists used to say that the only way fear and anxiety could be dealt with was through the brain, but now there are many of us who know that through the body we can relieve our anxieties and release the long pent-up tensions of hidden rage. We do this not through talk but through motion, through stretching and loosening our muscles.

The texture of a truly loose and relaxed muscle is viscous, somewhat like the white of a raw egg. When we are frightened or angry or are straining hard, our muscles are more like hard boiled eggs. We do not want to be raw-egg loose all the time, but we do need to be able to return to that state at will in order to erase the tensions of the past day or hours. We must find the right amount of muscular tension that we need to allow us to function most efficiently, whether it is the tension of a two-minute, a three-minute, or a four-minute egg. Likewise, ways must be found to relieve this tension.

Sorrow is like anger—it also must be faced. We need to weep as many bucket of tears as we have to shed, tears that contain anger, frustration, and self-pity, as well as love and the physical pain of separation. Relatives and friends who advise, "Forget the past, you must learn to live in the present," are well meaning, but they are not aware that emotions are also reflected in the body. The physical act of crying is muscular, as well as emotional. It takes many times longer for a muscle to be relaxed than for it to become tightened. Therefore, sometimes, many tears must be shed before we are relieved. When the last tear is truly shed we are increased in stature, strength and wisdom.

It takes courage to investigate our muscular tensions. I remember a pupil saying, "All my life I've been told to pull myself together, and here you are telling me to let myself go. What will happen to me if I do? I may be a monster inside."

It is true that we all have something of everything inside us, monsters as well as angels. However, when we gaze compassionately upon our monsters they lose their ferocity, become childlike, for they are that part of us that has not developed.

Aldous Huxley wrote that the way to our intuition is through our bodies, and the way to the spirit is through intuition. When fear, anxiety, rage and depression dwell in us, we hurt and we are blocked. We have no access to our inner selves, and life is dusty. Then, we spiral downward to entropy. One way we can reverse this spiral is through movement—stretching sore spots in our bodies, thinking of them, relaxing and comforting them, moving like seaweed flowing in the sea—becoming one with a natural rhythm.

My physician, a dear friend who took such good care of me during the years when I was so sick, tells me now that there is no trace of Lupus in my system. I feel certain that the constant emphasis on loosening the body—thirty years of repeating the relaxation ritual two or three times a week—must have had a lot to do with my improved health as well as my spirit.

Learning to concentrate on loosening muscles had helped me to learn to live one moment at a time, to learn to experience this second, for as Alan Watts said, "This second is eternity."[5] Over the years the world has become less dense, less solid. I remember clearly the first time I experienced a great revelation about space and movement. I was about seventeen.

My mother, my sister, and I were seated for lunch at our big square dining table. In front of me was a plate filled with *war bread,* a luscious food made with dark flour, molasses and raisins. This we had learned to make and eat as a patriotic gesture during World War I. And now, three years after the war's ending, I was reaching for a piece when my father joined us.

He apologized for being late but excused himself by saying that he had been reading a book that he could not put down, a book on astronomy by James H. Jeans (later Sir James Jeans).

"Do you realize," he said, helping himself to salad, "that all things, including us, are made of molecules?" We did. "But do you also realize that there is more space between each molecule than there are molecules?" "Furthermore," he went on, "all molecules are composed of atoms and there is more space between the atoms than there are atoms. Think about that," he said as he began to eat.

We thought about it and then my logical sister said, "If that is so, then when we wash dishes we are just dusting off space." We all laughed at that and I forgot to eat, thinking about space. I remember looking at the table, trying to imagine the great space within it. What I saw was the dark mahogany that father had rubbed with oil, an hour a day for an entire summer, until the wood glowed. I felt I should be able to see moving molecules in the wood's depth, but what I saw was the reflection of pale tea roses in a brass bowl in the center of the table. The knowledge that there was space, even in solid things, was exciting and important. When it turned out that atoms themselves are composed of particles, that whirl around their nuclei in the same manner as our planets whirl around the sun, it was obvious that the world was dancing.

All that stretching, moving, breathing, loosening, imagining is a path, a doorway, into a world that is only now beginning to be recognized. It is a world of probabilities where the hard lines between self and not-self are blurred or nonexistent, where there is a constant exchange of atoms and parts of atoms among all things in the universe.

If we live in such a universe, why are we holding on to our things, to our possessions, judging one another, condemning, fighting? How can we hold on to our fears when the only certainty is change? How can we hold on to our anger when, by moving, we can dispel it? When we spend our energies making ourselves miserable, do we dare to be joyous?

We are dancing—dancing—that is what being alive is—dancing! Of course, dancing may take the form of running, or walking, or moving slowly, or *imagining* ourselves running and dancing. Moving is aliveness and it is joy.

When I learned that the particles of which atoms are made are not made of *stuff* at all but are instead charges of energy, it became clear to me that all life, all living creatures, all plants, all trees, all growing things, as well as all rocks, stones and minerals are composed of moving, dancing particles of energy. I laughed out loud when I read in the *Tao of Physics* that:

> Modern physics has shown us that movement and rhythm are essential properties of matter: that all matter, whether here on Earth or in outer space, is involved in a continual cosmic dance.[6]

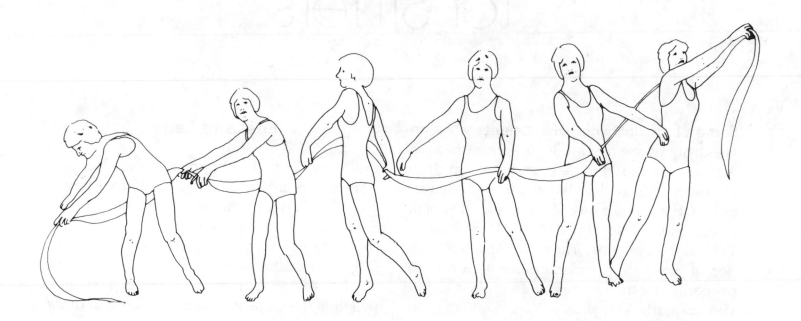

CHAPTER TWO

Recipes
for Sitters

Some of the following movements were devised many years ago, to prepare pregnant women for the delivery of their children. Therefore, it is evident that the movements are gentle. However, if any of them hurt, do not do them. Please do them NO MORE THAN TWICE the first time! Then increase the number of times slowly. Remember, you are not preparing for the Olympics. The aim is to give you comfort.

Feet and Legs

This is the first, most important place to begin working on our bodies. Your feet have served you well, have taken you many places, and are your friends. They may hurt sometimes, probably because they have been ill used.

It is the custom of our society for women to wear their legs encased in nylon stockings, which is the same as wrapping them in glass.

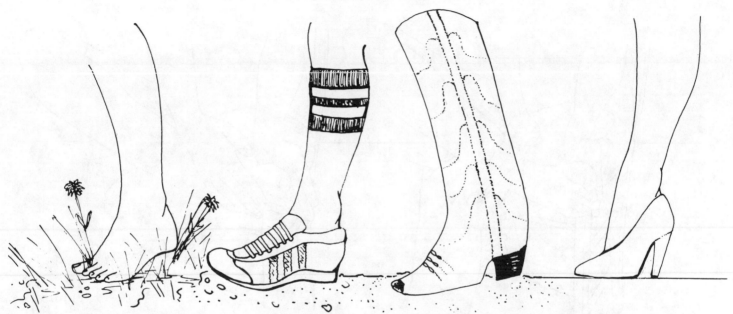

Both men and women tend to wear shoes that have very little resemblance to the shape of their feet.

All of us must walk on cement sidewalks. Cement is wonderful stuff—neat and tidy—but does not respond to our feet in the same way that the earth responds. If our feet are not stimulated, we tend to become lethargic and less interested in moving and in life. And life *is* movement. Primitive man walked barefoot on earth and rocks, grass and sand. His feet were accustomed to the feel of uneven surfaces; he walked up and down hills and mountains, over deserts and marshes. The nerves of his feet sent messages to him about textures and shapes, about gravity and his place on earth. Today, as we walk in our rigid shoes on hard flat pavements and soft flat carpets, we are separated from the earth. This robs us of vital energies.

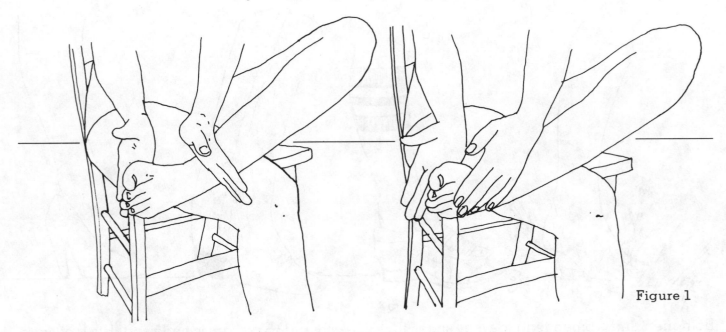

Figure 1

Patting the Feet

We can stimulate the nerves, as well as the circulation, by patting our feet:

Sit on your bed or chair and pull your left foot into your lap and pat it briskly but tenderly with both hands, the top as well as the bottom of the foot. **(Fig. 1)** It will soon feel warm.

Then pat your leg, patting all the way up to your hips. Give yourself a gentle spanking.

Now pat the right foot until it also feels warm.

Then pat your leg, all around, and up.

My 94-year-old friend, who could not reach her feet, found that a plastic fly-swatter was ideal for this job.

Foot Massage

With your left foot in your lap, hold it there with your left hand. With your right hand take hold of your big toe, move it forward and backward and around in a circle. **(Fig. 2a)** Hold it on each side of the toenail and pinch it just a little as you move it.

Figure 2a

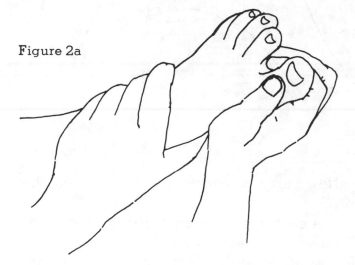

Now take hold of the next toe, pinching it gently and moving it back and forth and around in a circle. Do the same with your middle toe, your fourth toe and your little toe.

Still holding your foot, place the heel of your right hand on the ball of your left foot and curl your fingers over your toes. Now press your thumb into the arch of your foot, working around toward the ball of the foot. **(Figs. 2b and c)**

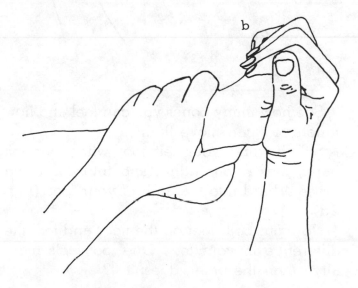

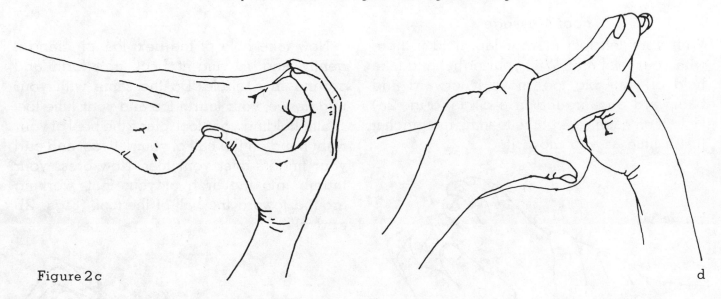

Figure 2 c   d

See how many bones you can feel and how much you can move them.

Still holding your left foot with your left hand, make your right hand into a fist and press it hard into the arch of your foot. **(Fig. 2d)**

Now put both feet on the floor and feel the difference in your feet. One foot feels more alive than the other, doesn't it?

Now pick up your right foot and repeat the process.

Move each toe back and forth and around.

Massage the metatarsal arch with your thumb.

Massage the arch of your foot with your fist.

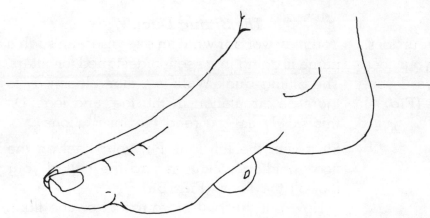

Figure 3

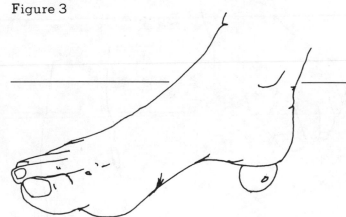

Ball Massage

Another massage for your feet: Use a small hard ball, about the size of a golf ball. Put it on the floor and roll your foot over it, pressing down so you can really feel it. **(Fig. 3)**

Be sure you roll your entire foot over the ball—toes, ball of the foot, arch and heel. When you find a sensitive place, press gently on that spot. See if you can work the pain out. Foot massage goes well with watching television.

Spread the Toes

See how far apart you can spread your toes. Try to move one toe at a time. Curl your toes under and then pull them back toward you. Wave your toes, slowly, then rapidly. **(Fig. 4)**

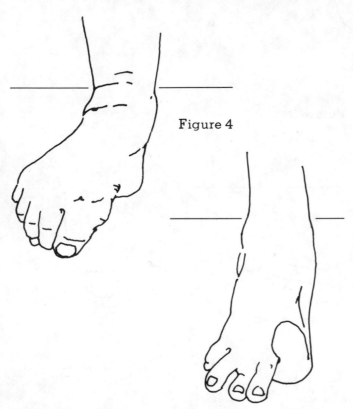

Figure 4

The Sitting Duck Walk

You may wonder what an exercise with such a name is doing in a section designed for sitters. The Sitting Duck Walk is a marvelous way to increase circulation in the feet and legs. Do this slowly as you read the instructions.

Start with the left foot. Put your heel on the floor, holding your toes and the ball of your foot off the floor. **(Fig. 5a)**

Now put the ball of your foot on the floor, raise your heel, keep toes still in the air. **(Fig. 5b)** Now put toes on the floor, with heel and ball off the floor. **(Fig. 5c)** Rest your left foot while you put the right heel on the floor, with right ball and toes in the air. Now put the right ball on the floor, with heel and toes in the air. Then toes on the floor with heel and ball in the air.

This sounds much more complicated than it is—you actually do it every day. This is the way we walk, but it happens too quickly and automatically to be aware of.

There is a Walking Duck Walk in the chapter for Walkers, but it is best to practice this maneuver while sitting, before you try it standing.

The Sitting Duck Walk

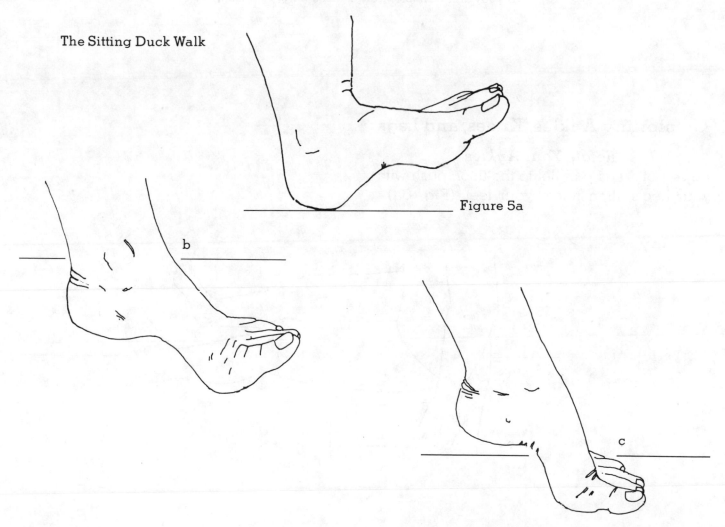

Figure 5a

b

c

Comforting Ankles, Knees, and Legs

Rotate Your Ankles

Raise both legs parallel to the floor; push with
your heels, then rotate your feet. **(Fig. 6a)**

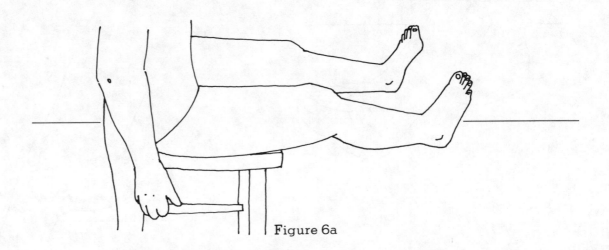

Figure 6a

Rotate inward so your toes touch, then point your toes down, then out so your heels are touching **(Figs. 6b and c)**, then up again and push with your heels. Go first one way and then the other.

Note: some people get cramps in the calf; if this happens to you, push with your heel. This will stretch the calf muscle.

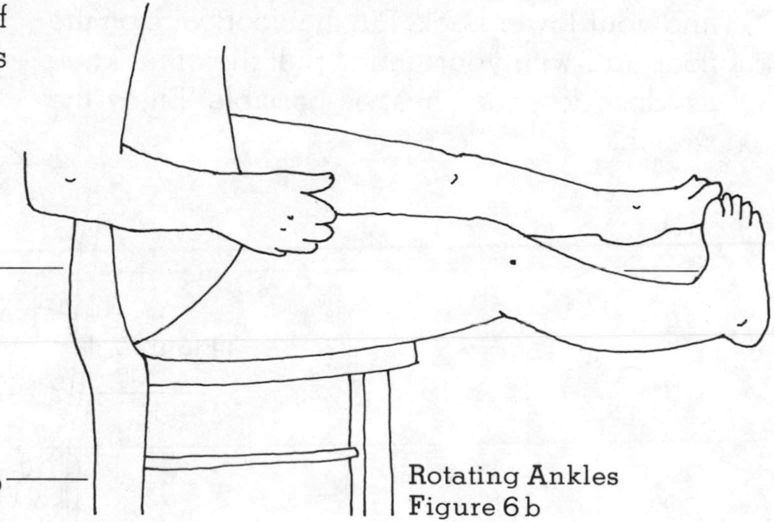

Rotating Ankles
Figure 6 b

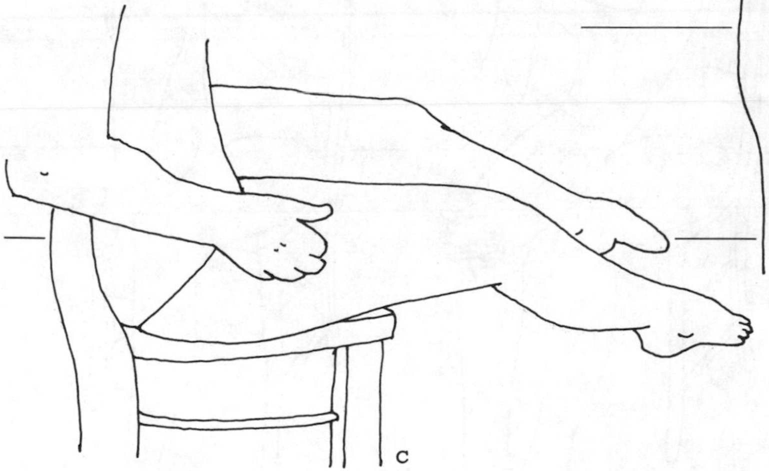

c

Knee to Chest

While still sitting on your chair, put both hands around one knee; with your hands pull your knee as close to your chest as you can. **(Fig. 7)**

Feel the stretch in your thigh, your buttocks and your lower back. Put that foot back on the floor and with your hands pull the other knee as close to your chest as possible. Enjoy the stretch.

Figure 7

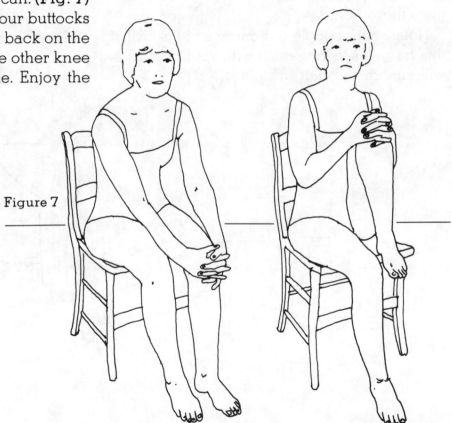

The Bounce: Tighten, Then Loosen, the Muscles You Sit On

The Bounce will help relieve your fatigue when you have to sit too long on a plane, on a bus, in church, in a waiting room, or in your own home. It will also strengthen the muscles of your buttocks and your lower back.

Put your hands under your buttocks on each side to guide your attention to the muscles your want to identify. Tighten, then loosen the buttocks muscles. This will cause you to rise up and down by a small but perceptible amount. The muscles of the buttocks will do this with no help from shoulders or arms.

If this seems silly or indecent, consider that you are strengthening your *gluteus maximus*, muscles that you need to climb hills and stairs and to move freely and vigorously. The movement not only strengthens these muscles, but gives rest to other muscles, bones, nerves and tissues in that area.

Once I worked in a retirement home that gave life care to its residents. One of them, confined to a wheelchair in the hospital section and who was both difficult and deaf, spent much of her time in the corridor near the nurses' station. Every time my duties took me to that part of the building she would yell loudly, "Mrs. Casper, my rectum hurts!" I would go to her and say, also loudly, "Mrs. Woods, tighten the muscles of your buttocks. Now let them go." "OH," she'd yell, "I feel better already."

Bending

This is a simple way to stretch and relieve tired muscles. Sit on an armless chair with feet and knees apart. Bend forward from the hips as far as possible, then sit straight. **(Fig. 8)**

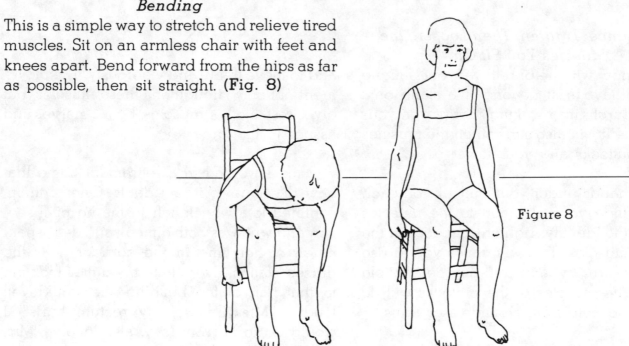

Figure 8

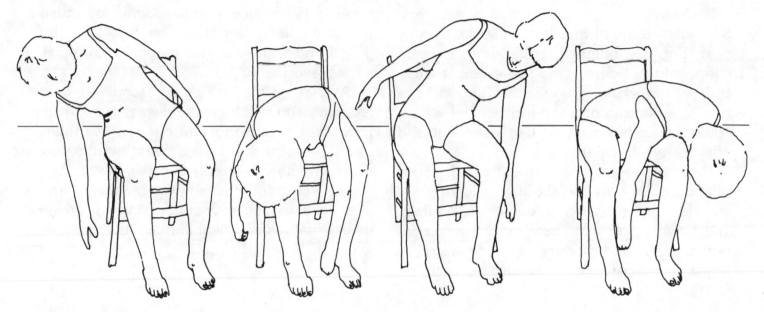

Figure 8 Bending

With head and torso facing front, bend sideways. See if your fingers can touch the floor. Bend first on one side, then the other. **(Fig. 8)**

Bend diagonally from the hips toward one knee. Sit up and bend diagonally toward the other knee. See how close to your knees you can reach with your chin. Sit up, then make a circle with your body. *Slowly* bend to the side, to one knee, to the front, to the other knee, to the other side and up. Reverse directions. *Go slowly* and be aware of how it feels.

I remember a pupil who was a secretary. She was pregnant and her back got awfully tired. She was relieved by bending, but said she would not dare to do these bends while she was working. I suggested she drop a pencil, an eraser, or her handkerchief, so she could stretch her back as she picked it up and thus relieve her pain.

The next week she came back to class giggling. She said that the day following our last class she dropped an eraser on the floor. The trouble was that she dropped it too enthusiastically and it bounced over toward her boss's desk. He jumped up and gallantly returned it to her. She tried the same ploy with a pencil on her other side. The boss saw the pencil and while she was reaching toward it, he retrieved it for her.

"At that point," she said, "I couldn't help laughing and told him what I was trying to do. Instead of being angry at me, he was interested. It seems that he has back trouble, too; that's why he's so cranky at times. I explained what I was doing and now we both bend and sway without tossing pencils and things on the floor. What his boss will think of this when he walks in, I can't imagine."

Rolling Your Spine

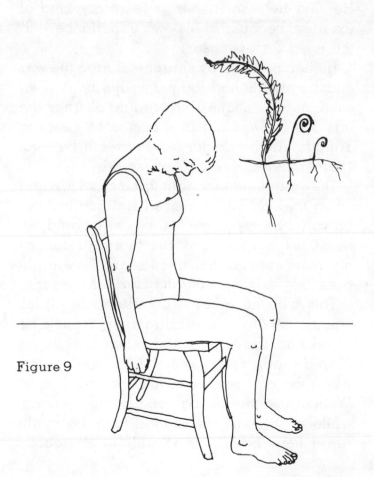

This is a different bend with different sensations. Sit straight in your chair. Let your chin sink down to your chest. Imagine you have lead on top of your head and let your head pull you downward, slowly, bone by bone.

Go as far as you can easily, then feel and be aware of the muscles holding you from going lower. Breathe deeply. Imagine your breath going into the tight spot so it will loosen. Then see if you can go down a little farther.

When you want to come up, slowly straighten your spine, bone by bone by bone from the bottom up. Unroll yourself like a fiddlehead fern from the bottom up. Think of each vertebra as your spine uncurls. **(Fig. 9)**

Figure 9

Tightening Muscles

You have many muscles you can tighten and relax at will. You have learned to tighten and relax your buttocks muscles and now let us see *how many muscles you can find* to tighten and release. Try these:

Tighten and relax the tops of your thighs. Tighten and relax the muscles of your upper arms. The calves of your legs. The insides and the outsides of your thighs. The bottoms of your thighs. See how many muscles you have control over.

It is refreshing when you are having enforced bed rest to tighten and relax all your muscles. It keeps them in good working condition and, most importantly, you are attending to your self, your body and your muscles, and they will thank you for it.

If muscles are not kept working and moving, they deteriorate. This was dramatically illustrated by a young man who brought his wife to one of my classes in preparation for childbirth.

He said he wanted her to learn my kind of exercise, because of his own experience with the need for exercise.

He had been hit by shrapnel during the war and fragments had lodged in his back. Two separate operations were required. After the first one he was put in a cast from knees to armpits. As the doctor left the room he said, "Remember to exercise every day."

The young man thought this a cruel jest and when the cast was removed six months later he could barely move his legs and could not stand. Six months of physical therapy returned his muscles to normal function and he was put back into a body cast after further surgery.

This time he understood. He spent all his time tightening and relaxing every muscle he could find. He tensed and relaxed while he played cards, read, or ate. After six months, when the cast was removed, he could walk! Without the muscle tightening and relaxing, while in the cast the second time, he might never have been able to walk at all again.

Side Twist

We've been tensing muscles for some time, so now let's start stretching them. **(Fig. 10)**

Sit in a straight armless chair. Take hold of the back of the chair on your left side with your left hand. Cross your right hand over your lap and take hold of the left side of the seat of your chair. Turn your torso to the left and twist around as far as possible.

Look at the floor in back of you, over your left shoulder. Alternate directions. Always twist in the direction of your hands, or you won't get anywhere. Always keep your buttocks and thighs straight ahead, or in the original position, as you twist.

You are stretching the muscles of your whole torso, as well as those of your neck and arms.

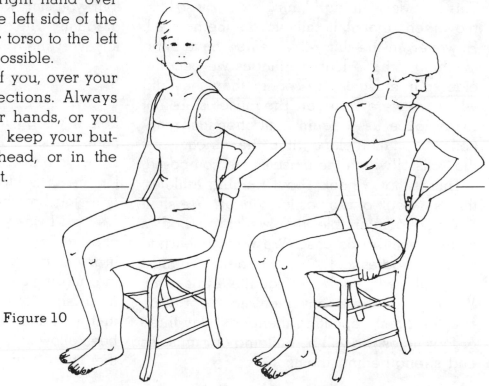

Figure 10

I want to warn you again that no matter how gentle these movements may seem, please *do them only once or twice* the first time. Do each movement slowly, and give it your complete attention, but do not do any movement more than twice until your muscles get used to it. This sounds as though I am giving you so little movement that it is silly to do them at all. However, in the thirty-five years I have been teaching, I have learned that as we become older our muscles tire sooner than they did when we were younger. The muscles are not ready to be used again until chemical reactions have taken place within the intricacies of the cells of which the muscles are composed.

This is not a book about training athletes; this is a book of recipes for *comfort.* We shall feel more comfortable when we use our bodies as they wish to be used. We want to learn to love our bodies, not to punish them. We must be gentle with ourselves—gentle and caring. When we do these movements, once or twice and then rest, repeating them next day three or four times, we will be building our muscles and strengthening them.

We are slower and cannot build muscles as rapidly as younger people, but we can do a lot to bring them up to their maximum performance. When you see instructions for exercises to be done twelve times, I would suggest that if you are near my age, which is seventy-four, you start with two and work up to twelve gradually. The gradual approach is really best for everyone.

Breathing

Before we go into more strenuous things, I think we should talk about breathing. Yes, I know you are breathing while you read this, for breath is life, but have you ever noticed *how* you breathe?

When I was young I was taught to raise my chest as I slurped in a noisy breath and pulled in my stomach. However, this kind of breathing allows you to use only a fraction of your lung capacity. My teachers had not realized that had the abdominal, or belly muscles, been allowed to relax and expand, as well as the chest muscles, there would have been room for much more air. Your lungs extend from the upper part of the rib cage to about the bottom of the ribs. The ribs are laced with muscles which allow them to expand and contract as you breathe, but the movement is limited. At the bottom of the lungs there are no bones to interfere with the expansion; there is instead a muscle, the diaphragm, which is dome shaped and attached to the ribs and backbone. When the belly muscles are relaxed, the full lungs push the diaphragm down, this pushes the organs of the abdominal cavity down which in turn push the belly *out*. This interaction cannot take place unless the belly muscles are *loose*.

Take a breath the way you usually do and notice where the air goes. Does it stop in your chest? Now try sticking your belly out and taking a breath. Did it feel different? Good.

Now just let your belly muscles be loose and take a deep breath. Did you notice that your belly expands automatically? It is as though you were filling a grocery bag; you put the first things in the *bottom* of the bag and fill the bag from the bottom up.

Think of your lungs as a grocery bag and the air as the groceries.

Practice taking a longer time pushing your air out than taking it in. For instance, if you breathe in through your nose to two counts, breathe out through your mouth to four counts; or if you breathe in for four counts, breathe out for eight. Then try giving a slight pause at the end of the inhale and again at the exhale.

Experiment with your breathing. For example, when you breathe out, blow outward with your mouth pursed as in whistling, slowing the release. Practice this when you are resting between exercises.

Swimming

Now let's do a movement that stretches other muscles of the upper part of the body as well as the middle. Let's go swimming. **(Fig. 11)**

Sit on the edge of your chair or bed. Lean forward as far as you can. Stretch one arm out forward as far as you can.
Now bring that arm back and push it out behind you while stretching the other arm forward.

Allow your body to turn from side to side as you extend your arms—you will be doing the crawl. Let your head stretch forward and turn with your body.

When you reach forward with your left arm, while your right arm extends behind you, your whole torso will turn to the right, just as it would do if you were swimming. And as your left arm comes back while your right arm extends, it is natural that you will turn to the left. Very gently stretch on one side and then the other, and then rest.

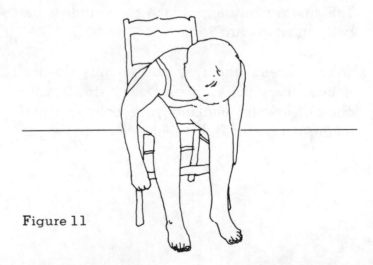

Figure 11

Now add another dimension to this movement: imagine you are swimming in clear delicious water in your favorite place—a river, a lake, the ocean, or wherever you have enjoyed swimming. You are stretching your arms, shoulders, neck and back and the water feels so good!

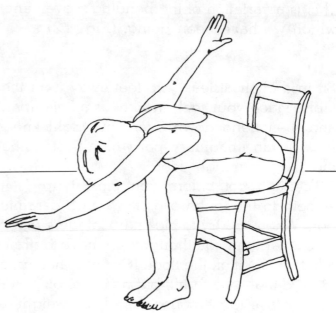

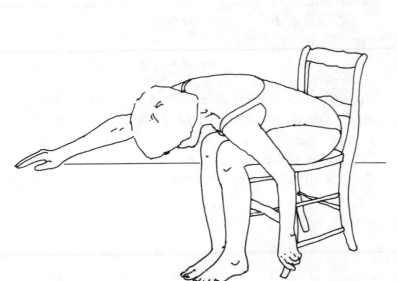

Figure 11 Swimming

Pick up Pots

This is a variation of the bending movements which we have been doing. **(Fig. 12)**

Sit in a chair at least two feet away from the table. Place your feet and knees a little apart and then bend down over your right knee. Pick up an imaginary pot which is standing there by your right foot.

Feel the pot before you pick it up. Is it smooth to the touch or is it a rough ceramic pot? When you try to pick it up imagine that it is heavier than you thought; you have to strain a little to get it off the floor. It is not so heavy as to be dangerous to lift, but heavy enough for you always to be conscious of the weight.

Pick it up slowly; be aware of your back as it straightens. Bring the pot up chest-high, where you can look at it. Then reach to put it on a very high shelf to your left. You will have to stretch your back and your arms and even your fingers to get it up there.

Now sit back and rest and breathe with your belly loose, letting air flow into every corner of your lungs. Rest a few minutes; then reach down to your left foot, find your pot, feel it, lift it slowly as before, and put it on a very high shelf to your right, stretching all the way. Sit back and breathe.

This time reach down and find your pot directly in front of you, between your feet. It is really heavy. When it is at eye level, look at it carefully. It is ugly. Lift it up to a high shelf directly above your head. Start to put it on the shelf, but stop, consider: this is an ugly pot, it is heavy because it contains all your troubles. So, instead of putting it away, dash it onto the floor with all your strength.

Figure 12 Picking up Pots

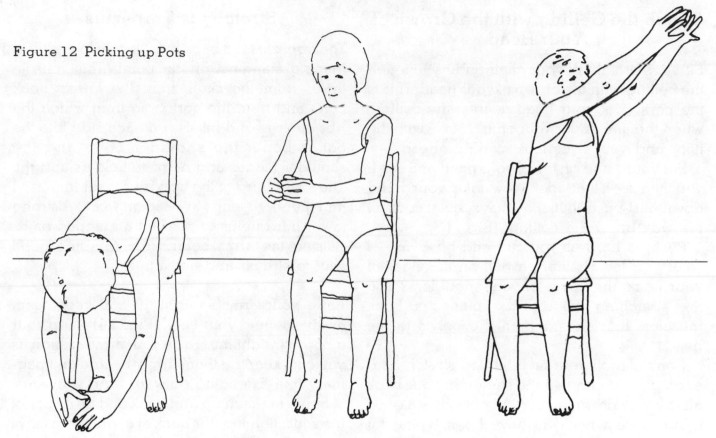

Touch the Ceiling with the Crown of Your Head

Sit very straight in your chair and try to touch the ceiling with the crown of your head. This is the portion of your head nearest the ceiling, when the line under your chin is level with the floor and your eyes look straight ahead.

Put your hand on top of your head and see if you can feel that spot. Now take your hand down and push that spot, that special spot, all the way up to the ceiling. (**Fig. 13**)

Push as hard as you can and be aware of what you feel. Is there a pull on the sides of your neck, the backs of your shoulders? You are stretching the *erectus spinae*, or back muscles, that extend from the pelvis to the head.

Don't clench your teeth. If you stretch hard enough, you can feel the stretch in your back all the way down to your buttocks. It is a good thing to do when you have been typing for some time, or driving a car, or sewing. It keeps you from getting kinks.

Stretch the Trapezius

The *trapezius* is a back muscle that looks like a triangle standing on its point. This muscle arises from the skull, from the lowest neck bone and from the vertebrae from which the ribs emerge and inserts on each side into the collar bone, the shoulder bone and the shoulder blades and helps to hold us upright. The lower third of the trapezius is seldom used and therefore tends to become weak. A strong lower third helps to prevent a humped back. Raising the arms behind the ears is a good way to stretch and activate it.

Raise your arms straight up and keep them always behind your ears. (**Fig. 14**) Keep your elbows straight and raise your arms as high as you can, keeping them firmly behind an imaginary line extending outward from your ears.

Strive to reach up and back and be aware of the sensation in your back at about the base of your ribs. This is the lowest point of the trapezius.

Please be very careful about how much you do this stretch. Since so few of us ever pick apples or cherries, or swing from branches, the muscle is tender and needs to be developed very slowly or it may hurt—a lot.

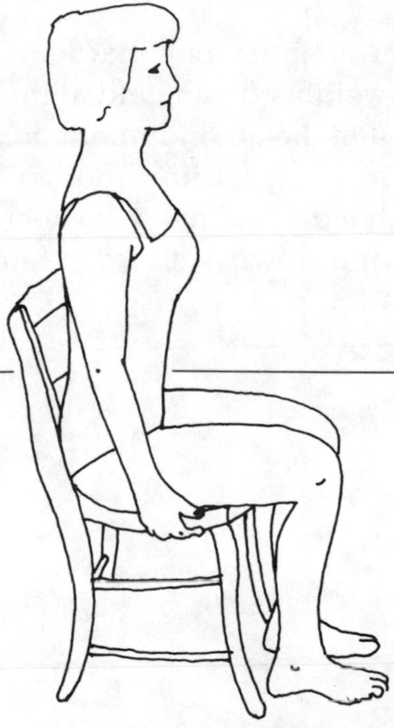

Figure 13
Touch the Ceiling

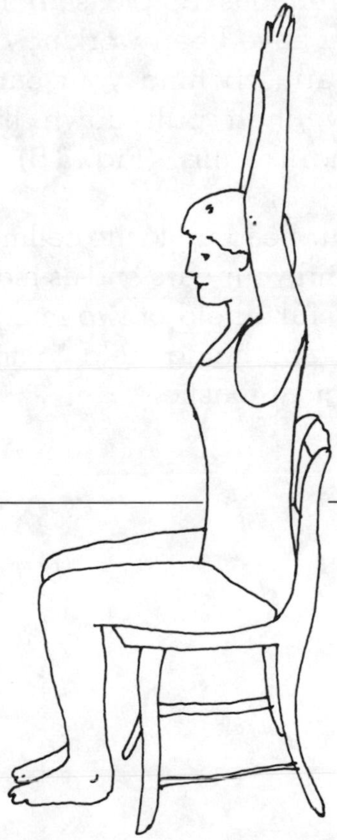

Figure 14
Stretch the Trapezius

Pulling and Pushing Down the Weight

This is a continuation of the last two movements and is quite strenuous. So please don't do it right now, if you have been working on trying to raise your arms behind your ears. Rest until tomorrow, then pull down the weight, which is done like this. **(Fig. 15)**

Push the crown of your head up to the ceiling. Raise your arms behind your ears and as high as you can get them. Take hold of two imaginary weights which are being held to the ceiling by some magical elastic.

Pull the weights down to your chest. Now push them down to the floor. Hold this posture long enough to be aware of how it feels, then relax, breathe and rest. Don't do this more than once or twice at a time.

You must pull hard and slowly to pull the weights down, and at the same time be aware that the ceiling might come down also, so you must sit tall in order to hold it up with your head. You need to push up with your head and down with your hands and fingers.

Figure 15
Pulling and Pushing Down the Weight

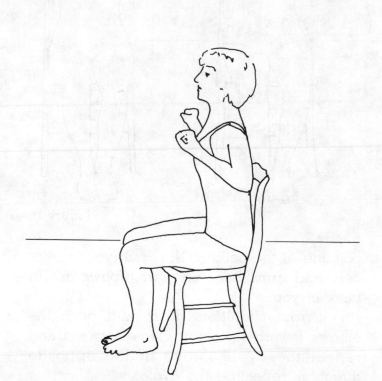

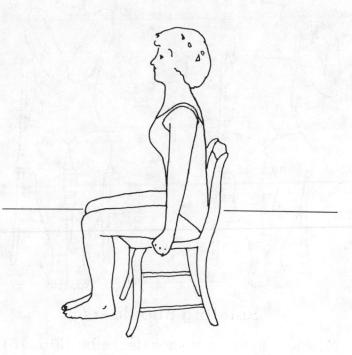

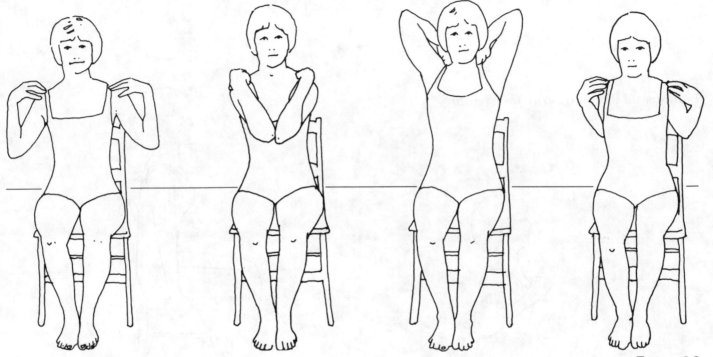

Figure 16

Rotating Shoulders

Now let's limber our shoulders a bit. **(Fig. 16)** Put the tips of the fingers of your left hand on your left shoulder and the tips of the fingers of your right hand on your right shoulder.

Bring your shoulders forward so your elbows can touch in front of you. Raise your shoulders and arms so that your elbows are pointing at the ceiling. Now pull your shoulders and arms back so your elbows are in back of you.

Pull your shoulders down and push the elbows toward the floor. Come forward and repeat the cycle. Move in the opposite direction, repeating the cycle.

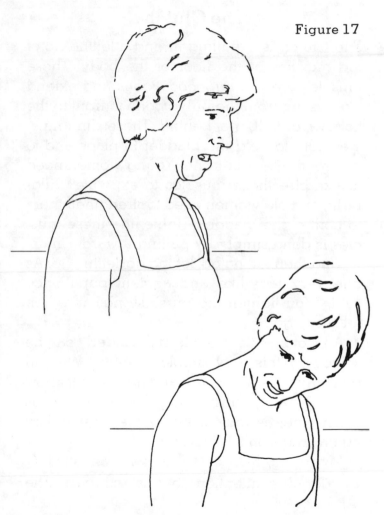

Figure 17

Rolling Heads

Now is the time for heads to roll. **(Fig. 17)** Be very loose. Let your jaw drop. Let your head hang forward.

Slowly roll your head to one side.
Let your head drop and roll it to the other side. Pretend that your head is a block of wood floating on the bay, swaying gently from side to side.

Now slowly roll the head up on one side, then toward the front, until your neck is straight and eyes are looking straight ahead. Continue the circle down to the other shoulder, then forward.

Reverse directions. Remember to be loose. If you feel a tight spot, stop and think about it and breathe into that spot. It will help to loosen the tight muscle. Continue, remembering to reverse directions.

The Clutch

The Clutch is a pulling-in and a letting-go of the muscles of the floor of the body. These muscles are the *pubococcygeus* and extend like a sling from the pubic bone in front to the *coccyx*, or tailbone, behind. These sling muscles help to hold the bladder in place and to control the flow of urine. Young women need to exercise these muscles to expedite childbirth, and old women need to strengthen them to control the bladder. Tightening these muscles is done simply by pulling inward—in, in, in, and then letting go, letting go, letting go. As one very lady-like and ancient pupil once said, "You tighten the purse strings and then let them go."

A lot of bladder trouble of the elderly can be solved by this very simple exercise. We can do it any time, anywhere and no one will know what we are doing. Pull in and release as many times as you can easily, then rest and try again. But don't forget it.

My friend, MK, saved herself from surgery by rigorous attention to this exercise. The doctor told her that her bladder was actually slipping out, the muscles were too weak to hold it in place. So she pulls in and releases hundreds of times a day and her bladder is back where it should be with no surgery needed.

Hands and Fingers

Our hands do a great deal for us but we scarcely bother with them except to keep them clean and manicured. If you've noticed that your hands are a little stiff in the morning and don't work quite so well as they did, spend some time gently massaging them, with love.

Massage them while you are in the bathtub or while holding them in a bowl of warm water, being careful to see that each joint moves. Find the places that are sore and move them slowly, gently. Then try the following movements. **(Fig. 18)**

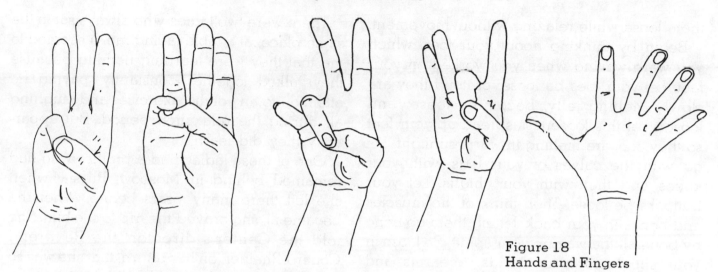

**Figure 18
Hands and Fingers**

Cross your thumb and little finger with your thumb on the outside. Now cross them so your thumb is on the inside. Cross them back and forth, thumb and little finger, several times.

Cross thumb and fourth finger, then thumb and middle finger and then first finger. Now stretch your fingers as far apart as you can, then gently shake them out. Make figure eights with your hands, moving them from the wrist with the fingers loose.

My ninety-four year old friend, MK, has bought herself some jacks. She sits on the floor and plays jacks, using first her right hand, then her left hand. This amuses her and exercises her arthritic fingers.

Loosening

You have tightened or stretched many of the muscles in your body while just sitting, so now let us try to think of these muscles and let them loose while relaxing without movement.

Begin by thinking about your toes, which you were waving when you worked on your feet. Let your toes be loose; pretend they are slowly melting jelly, becoming looser and looser. Let this looseness spread up your feet so they, too, are melting in warm sunlight. Let go with the calves of your legs, with your knees and then with your thighs. Let your buttocks be loose. Then think of the muscles and bones in your back, letting them go bone by bone all the way up your spine. Be loose in your shoulders, your hands, forearms and upper arms. Let go at the back of your neck, let your jaw drop, let your tongue be loose, let your eyelids close and just let go all over. Now yawn and stretch leisurely; then get up very slowly.

In 1963 I taught at a senior center where sixty or seventy people gathered around long tables for lunch and recreation and fifteen or twenty minutes of exercising before settling down to the main business most of them had come for, namely, bingo.

There were two ladies who always sat in the same place, at a table facing me. It seemed to me that they were learning nothing because they talked together constantly, paying no attention to any of the exercises and laughing all during the relaxation period. But apparantly they did learn.

One of these ladies had a brother who had remained behind in Moscow, Russia, when she left there many years before. When he became ill, she braved the trip to see him. She told the Center's director, the Reverend Conard Rheiner, on her return, that she was so terrified of traveling that she didn't move once from her seat on the plane and was too afraid to get off during the London stopover. He asked her if she had not been too stiff to move at the end of the long flight. She said no, because she had done her exercises. She moved her feet and legs, tightened her buttocks, stretched her back and her neck, twisted, turned, and relaxed when she needed sleep. She did this halfway round the world and back, and it made me realize, again, the value of these exercises.

CHAPTER THREE

Recipes for Movers

I hope those of you who feel you cannot get down on the floor will read this chapter and eventually have the courage to try some of these movements. Before you say, "If I get down on the floor, I'll never get up again," read the next instruction, please.

How to Get up Off the Floor

Get down on the floor and stretch out on your back as though you had fallen. Now roll over on one side. Bend the knee nearest the floor. **(Fig. 19a)**

Slowly push yourself into a sitting position, using your arms and hands to do so. From this position it will be easy to get on your hands and knees. **(Figs. 19b and c)**

Now put your right foot flat on the floor. Put both hands on your right thigh and push down on that thigh and up you will come. **(Figs. 19d and e)**

If your left side is stronger, put your left foot on the floor and push on your left thigh.

Figure 19 How to Get up Off the Floor

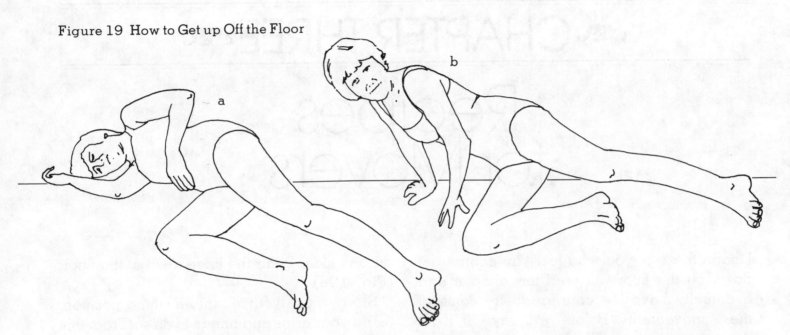

I wish everyone knew this trick because so many older people are afraid they can never get up off the floor if they fell.

Lilly, a slight woman whom I judged at first to be sixty, asked, the first time she came to class, if she could do the exercises on a chair instead of getting on the floor. I said she could, but asked why. She said she couldn't get up from the floor. So I showed her this maneuver, and she became a happy member of the class.

Later I learned that she had come to class in desperation because her children were pressuring her to move into a retirement home where residents ate in a common dining room and did no cooking themselves. Lilly had fallen once, and only because a neighbor had

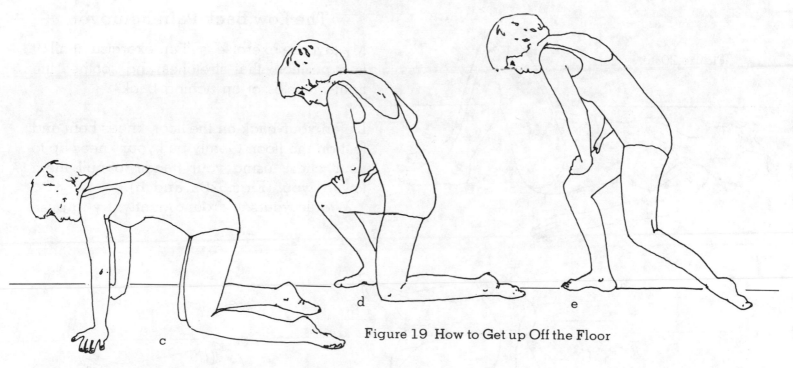

Figure 19 How to Get up Off the Floor

heard her cries for help had she been able to get up again. This frightened her children, as it frightened her.

"But I don't want to give up my home," she said. "I like to have parties, to invite my grandchildren and their friends. I cook great meals for them so they like to come to my house. You cannot expect young people to enjoy visiting an invalid grandmother. Now I demonstrate, to everyone who will watch, how to get up off the floor, and my children have stopped pestering me. You see," she smiled, "though I'm well over eighty I am not helpless."

The Low Back Pain Remover

My favorite exercise isn't an exercise at all. It is a position, that stretches and soothes the tight muscles of an aching back.

Lie on your back on the floor, knees bent and feet on the floor. Gently pull your knees up to your chest, using your hands to pull them toward you. **(Figs. 20a and b)**

Wiggle yourself around gently; try to push

Figure 20 a

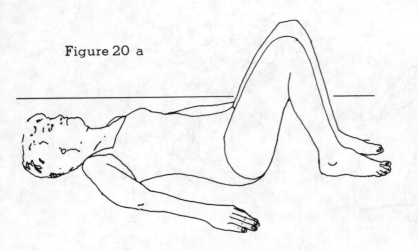

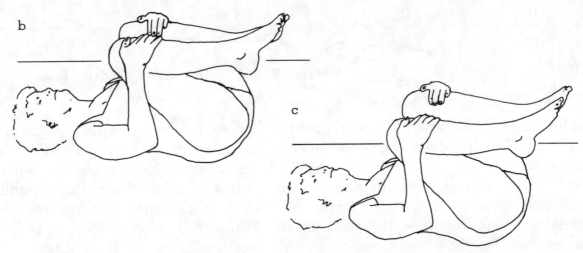

b

c

the bones of the small of the back into the floor. Let your knees fall back toward your feet.

Pull your knees to your chest again while allowing them to spread apart so that they can get closer to you. **(Fig. c)**

Become extremely conscious of the bones of your back as they dig into the floor during this exercise. Feel your *sacrum* (the solid bone of the lower spine) on the floor when you release your knees. Be aware of the *spinous processes* of your vertebrae as you pull your knees toward you.

Think loose, let the back muscles be loose, loose, loose. Let this looseness sink in, way into your being, so there is no tightness anywhere.

As you think loose, know that you are straightening the curve of the lower back where sometimes a lot of pain lies. This straightening requires very little effort but does require a great deal of *non* effort.

We all have an interior muscle, the *psoas*, that stabilizes the pelvis, holding the posterior down. However, the *erector spinae*—a group of muscles extending from the pelvis to the skull—are a counter balance for the psoas. When they are in tight contraction they tend to pull the posterior up, which can cause a swayback and be very painful.

These back muscles seem very responsive to fear. I imagine that when we lived in the jungle and thought we saw a tiger in the bush, these erector muscles tightened immediately, readying us to throw a weapon or run like the wind.

Today when anything threatens us, the muscles of the back, including the muscles of the buttocks and the anus and those extending all the way up to the shoulders and the neck, tend to tighten. When this tension, of which we are unaware, continues over a period of time, we hurt.

So what we need to do now is to comfort and release the tense muscles of the back by lying with our knees to our chest and thinking... loose...loose...loose.

Figure 21

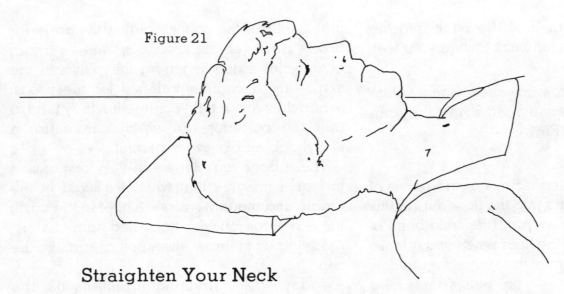

Straighten Your Neck

When we were young, we could lie on the floor with only a very slight space between the neck and the floor. But now, at seventy-four, I can put my whole fist between the floor and my neck.

How did this happen? How is it with you? I suppose, because there have been periods of non-attention, periods of not caring for my body and also because of age, the beautiful elegant articulation of my body has gotten out of balance; and no longer functions perfectly. So, instead of moaning because I am imperfect, I shall take a book, between one and one-half and two inches in thickness, and use it to hold my head.

Place the book so that the hump at the back of your head will rest upon it. **(Fig. 21)**

Be sure that your head is on the edge of the

Raise Your Arms Above Your Head

book so that only the hump rests on the book. This position allows the neck to straighten.

Straightening the neck this way feels good. Try it. You may need to experiment to find a book just the right height for you. When it feels right, it's helpful to place a book beneath the head for all the floor exercises, including the Low Back Pain Remover.

If using a book is uncomfortable for you, forget it. We are all different and must find what seems right for us individually. Listen to your body; accept what it tells you.

Lie on the floor with knees bent, feet flat on the floor. Move your arms on the floor until they are above your head. Go slowly. Keep your entire arm on the floor. Return the arms to your starting position.

If you find that your elbow has left the floor, stop and start over. Raise your arms only as far as they can go comfortably, while keeping them on the floor. Then try again tomorrow, and tomorrow, and the day after that. It may take some time to stretch out tight muscles that haven't stretched that way for a long time.

The Bridge

This is a modification of a yoga posture that I adapted years ago to meet the needs of pregnant women, who often have low back pains. It's a gentle exercise.

Lie on your back. Place your feet flat on the floor, about twelve inches apart. Press down on your heels as you raise your buttocks off the floor. Raise them as high as you comfortably can. **(Fig. 22)**

Weight is now resting on your heels, shoulders and upper part of your back. Start lowering yourself, coming down so that the vertebra bone nearest your shoulders reaches the floor first, then the next bone, the next one and then the next. Feel each bone as it pushes into the floor.

As you raise your buttocks, feel the stretch in your back. As you lower your body and reach the bone that is in the curve of the swayback, see if you can push that bone into the floor. To do this you will have to lengthen your back by pushing your buttocks forward. Wag your tail so you can feel that bone, and then the next and the next until your back is hugging the floor.

Imagine that your back is a bolt of silk—that has been rolled out, smooth and shining. Rest and breathe. At first you may find it difficult to press parts of your back down, but once the muscles loosen you will enjoy it.

Figure 22

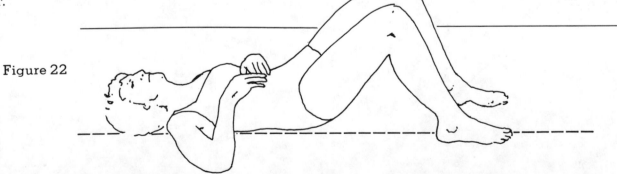

The Neck Stretch

After you have done the Bridge a couple of times, remain on your back with your knees bent and your feet flat on the floor.

Put your hands behind your head—not at the nape of the neck, but on the bulge (*occipital*) of the head, clasping your fingers to hold it comfortably.

Raise your head with your hands as far off the floor as possible, using your arms, hands and shoulders, assisted by your belly muscles. The point is not to sit up, but to get the head, neck and, if possible, the shoulders away from the floor. Now relax your neck and belly muscles and allow your arms and hands to hold your head off the floor. **(Fig. 23)**

The weight of your head is supported by your hands, not held up by your stomach muscles. Your neck is completely relaxed; your jaw is loose. Start lowering your head, slowly.

Your hands are gently stretching your neck longer while lowering the upper part of your body, bone by bone. Try to feel the vertebrae as each separate bone meets the floor. When your head is all the way down on your book (if you are using one), gently remove your hands and enjoy the sensation.

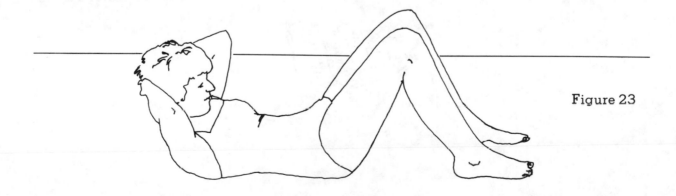

Figure 23

Twisting Spiral Stretch

Remain on your back with knees bent and feet flat on the floor. Stretch your arms out so your body forms a cross. Put your *right* leg, bent, over your left leg. Let both legs slowly fall to the *right.*

Go in that direction as far as you can with ease, while still keeping your shoulders on the floor. Feel where you are stretching and be aware of the muscles which prevent your legs from going nearer to the floor.

Think of these spots as you do the stretch, take a breath, and imagine you are sending air to them, breathing into them. You may find that your legs are now nearer to the floor because some of the tense muscles have relaxed.

Come back to starting position. Put your *left* knee over your right knee and let your legs fall to the *left.* See how far they fall, then breathe into the spots which are holding them from falling farther. Do this only twice, then rest.

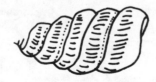

Spiral with Straight Legs

As you become looser and looser, and have discovered how many muscles you can stretch in the spiral position, straighten your legs and, if you have room on the floor, try this.

Swing your right leg over toward your left side. Try to put your right foot into your left hand (without bending knee or elbow). **(Fig. 24)**

Do it easily but stretch as far as you can, pausing to feel the stretch, to breathe, to send air to the tense muscles.

Repeat with the other leg. Now pull your knees up to your chest and rest.

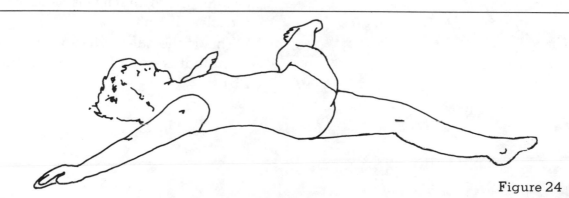

Figure 24

Raise and Lower *One* Leg

Warning: There is one exercise you may have expected, but which you will not find in this book. That is the dreadful, strenuous, the hard-on-your-back exercise in which you raise both legs vertical to the floor then lower them with your legs straight. Please, please, please do not do that!

Some very strong people, who have strong backs and who have done it all their lives, can handle it. But, for most of us, it puts a strain on our backs that we should not endure. The effort of lowering our legs is injurious because this means that our back must arch off the floor. We thus are tightening the muscles that gave us a sway-back in the first place—and what we want to do is stretch and relax them.

There are people who have badly damaged their backs doing this exercise. They thought, as many have, that it was good for the stomach muscles. It isn't.

This is the safer way to do a similar movement that *is* good for stomach muscles. **(Fig. 25)**

Lie on your back, knees bent, feet flat on the floor. Raise and straighten your right leg so it is vertical. Press into the floor with your left heel. Keep your left knee bent. Make sure your back is flat. Slowly lower your right leg. Do the same procedure with your left leg.

By putting your hands on your abdomen, you can feel how the stomach muscles are being contracted. You can watch the movement of your hands and know what your *rectus abdominus* (the strong muscle covering the belly) is doing.

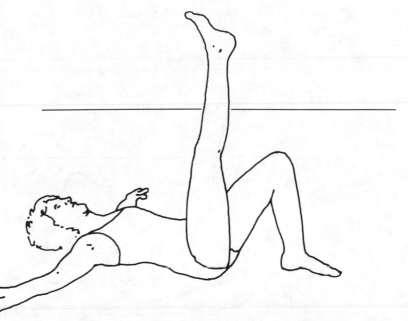

Figure 25 Raise and Lower One Leg

Ann's Favorite

Ann has a very flat stomach, and this is what she does every day to maintain it. **(Fig. 26)**

Lie on your back, knees bent, feet and back flat on the floor, arms at your sides. Raise your *right* leg above your head. Raise your *left* arm in the same way at the same time.

Lower your right leg and your left arm to their starting position. Raise your *left* leg and your *right* arm; then lower.

Do this two or three times the first day and add one time each day.

If this produces any soreness in the abdominal wall, rest a day and then go back to the beginning, doing it only once or twice. Go *slowly*, and end by bringing knees to chest to rest.

Strenuous exercise breaks down muscle tissues, which are repaired during rest. Muscles become stronger through this process of breakdown and repair if enough time is allowed for rebuilding. The trouble is that those of us who are over fifty, sixty,

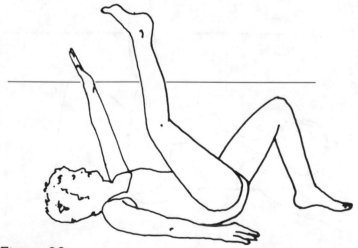

Figure 26

seventy, or eighty, do not repair our tissues as rapidly as younger people. This means that when we exercise too much, we may be destroying our tissues instead of building them.

So, if you are over sixty and hear about an exercise you like, do it once or twice and then stop. If the instructions are to start doing it ten times and work up to fifty, you're to start with two times and work up to ten.

The Angry Cat, Happy Puppy, Lazy Donkey

Lie on your back with your knees brought up to your chest. Roll over on your side and get on your hands and knees. Your knees should be about a foot to a foot and a half apart and so should your hands. Arms and elbows are straight.

Think of the spot in the center of the curve of the small of the back, the swayback. This is the spot you were sensing while you were doing the Bridge. Put a hand there, see if you can find it. When you have found it, remove your hand and try to push that spot up to the ceiling. You are an angry cat! **(Fig. 27a)**

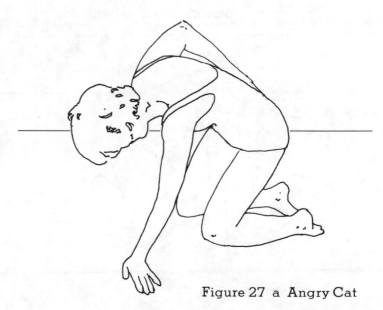

Figure 27 a Angry Cat

Arch your back as high as it will go. Wag your tail. Let your buttocks wag back and forth. You are now a happy puppy. **(Fig. 27b)**

Now let your back sway down so you look like a lazy donkey. **(Fig. 27c)**

Do this a few times. Arch your back and sit back on your heels. Put your head down on the floor and rest. The farther apart your knees are, the more comfortable you will be.

This is not just a child's game. It is one version of the Pelvic Rock, which changes the relationship between the pelvis and the spine. Sense this difference. See if you can become acutely aware of the difference between the donkey and the cat positions. You can practice this movement while lying on your side, or back, in bed. Soon, we will learn to do this rocking movement while standing, so, please, practice it now.

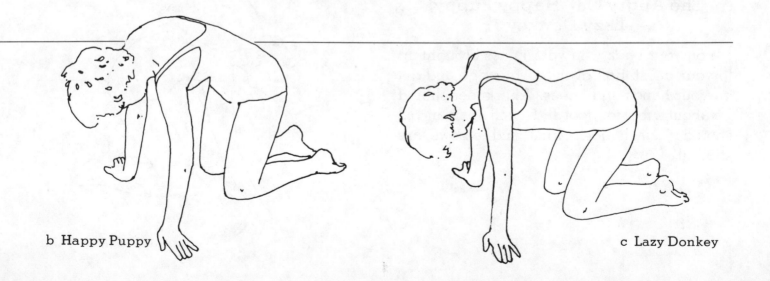

b Happy Puppy   c Lazy Donkey

Crawling

Now—get on your hands and knees and crawl! It's easy to do—though a little strenuous, so don't do it very long. Crawl slowly, stretching one arm out in front of you as far as you can, while bringing the opposite knee forward as far as you can. **(Fig. 28)**

Crawl the way a child crawls. When the right hand goes forward, the left knee follows. Can you feel what is happening to your back muscles?

Be aware of the movement and stretching in those muscles. You are strengthening them as a child strengthens her muscles. At the same time your are training yourself, as she does, so that you will be able to walk easily in a contralateral fashion: left leg steps as right arm swings, right leg steps as left arm swings.

It has been found that babies who do not have the opportunity to crawl sometimes have developmental difficulties such as dyslexia, difficulty in reading, a unilateral walk, or other physiological problems. It has also been found

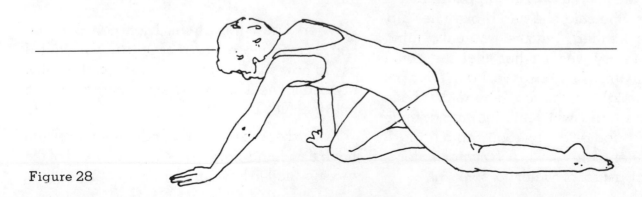

Figure 28

that a person with such a difficulty can sometimes be helped by returning to the stage of crawling, temporarily, no matter what the age of the person might be. It appears necessary for the human body to go through certain stages of development—crawling is one of them.

Crawling also aids the memory, by bringing blood to the head. I have found it helpful to crawl a bit when I can't remember something important.

Crawling as a means of locomotion is illustrated by this story. I volunteered my services to teach in a newly opened retirement home. The group was small and changed from week to week. One day a woman appeared in a wheelchair. She said she had broken her hip, which was healing, but the traumatic thing about this injury was, for her, that she could not take a bath. "Just because I can't yet put my whole weight on this leg," she said, "I have to stay in bed and wait until the nurses' aide has time to come to my room and bring a basin of water to my bed. A *basin* of water— ugh! I want a *tub* of water to soak in!"

I assured her all would be well eventually. In the meantime, she could strengthen the rest of her muscles by doing the movements for sitters with the group. Finally I knew the rest of the class needed a different kind of movement, so I asked the wheelchair lady to watch while the rest of us got down on the floor and did the Angry Cat and Happy Puppy movement. Then we crawled. The wheelchair lady had been watching the crawling closely, when, to my consternation, she slipped out of her wheelchair and crawled happily down the hall. I was terrified—but she returned, laughing, and crawled up into her wheelchair then wheeled herself away, thanking me for the fun.

When I saw her again, I learned that she had a good tub every morning now. When I asked how she did it she said, "I just slip out of my bed to the floor, crawl to the bathroom and into the tub. It's easy."

A word about bathtubs: I hope that all of you have firm hand-holds to help you get out of the tub, no matter how strong or limber you are.

Ride a Horse

Stand with your feet well apart, toes pointing straight ahead. Stand loosely. Now simply bend your knees up and down as though you were riding a horse. **(Figs. 29a and b)**

When you ride a horse, you move gently up and down. Remember—you are riding a gentle horse, not a bucking bronco. Let yourself swing a little from side to side. Let your hips swing gently, too. Be aware of how good it feels when your pelvis is allowed to be free. Let your hips make a gentle circle. Some people feel embarrassed and self-conscious when they begin these motions, so do it in private until you feel easy about it.

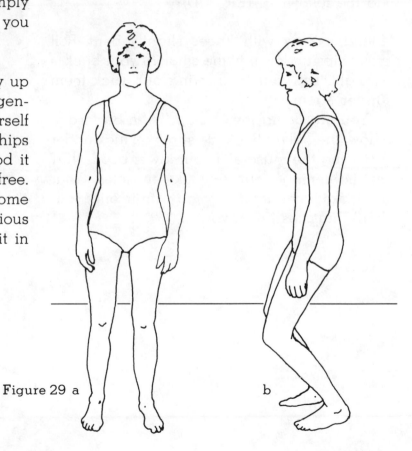

Figure 29 a   b

The Standing Pelvic Rock

Once your pelvis is free and can move easily, do the following. **(Fig. 30)**

Stand loosely with knees slightly bent. Roll your hips under until the small of your back is straight. Let your hips swing out. Tuck them under again.

You are doing the "bumps" of a burlesque show, the Pelvic Rock. Be sure you tuck under by using the muscle of your lower back, NOT by tightening your buttocks muscles. Your buttocks have nothing to do with it, only your back muscles are involved.

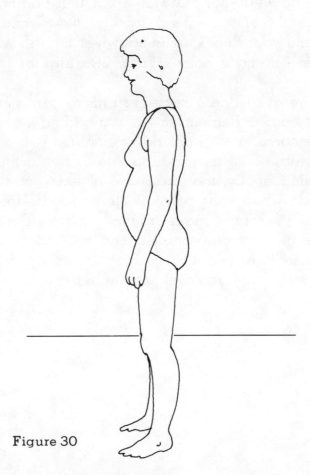

Figure 30

Every time I do the Pelvic Rock I think of Maggie, a white-haired, big-bosomed, imposing lady in her sixties who came to me in distress thirty years ago because of a back problem. She could walk, but could not stand for more than three minutes without unbearable pain in her lower back. She had lived with this affliction for several years, as no doctor seemed to know how to help her, but now was a time of crisis and she needed help.

"My son is getting married," she said dramatically.

"This is a crisis?" I asked, thinking she needed a psychiatrist.

"It's wonderful, his marriage: he's forty years old and we were afraid he'd never make it. The problem is that he has chosen the only child of a very rich and social family and the wedding will be big. They've sent out five hundred invitations and I will have to stand in the receiving line for hours, and I can't do it."

She was almost weeping.

"My husband says he will take me in a wheelchair and my doctor says he will put me in the hospital, but I want to be there on my own two feet just like anybody else."

"All right," I said, "We've got four weeks to get rid of your swayback. Get down on the floor."

So she learned how to pull her knees to her chest, and to rock and stretch the tight muscles of her back. She learned to lie on the floor with her legs on her bed (I'll tell you about this at the end of this chapter), and she learned to rock her pelvis. Maggie hooted with laughter when I first showed her this movement, but I told her she had better learn how to do it, as it would be her life saver. After the wedding she came to tell me about it.

"It was a wonderful wedding," she said. "I looked very elegant in a flowered velvet chiffon dress and a picture hat. I stood in the receiving line, and as I extended my hand and said, 'How do you do, Mrs. Smith,' I'd slowly tuck my hips under and when I said, 'How nice to see you, Mr. Smith,' I'd let them go. Nobody knew what I was doing except my husband, who was grinning all afternoon. Of course he was pleased with the marriage, but he was even more tickled with me. Nothing hurt. We had a wonderful time."

When you are standing in line, or waiting for a bus, and your back begins to hurt, try the same movement. Ever so gently, and slowly, loosen your knees, tuck your hips under, then let them go. It will relieve the pain and fatigue in your lower back. Do it slowly. No one will notice.

The Squat

Helene and Julian lived at the foot of my hill in 1949. We were friends who saw each other occasionally. Then Helene got pregnant and joined my class in "Preparation for Motherhood."

One day, when we had been working on the back and its relation to hips and head, Helene said that Julian had been complaining that his back hurt.

"He's so stubborn. He won't go to a doctor— he just complains. Do you think you could help him?"

I was only forty at the time and had not learned that only fools rush in before they are invited. So I said that I'd be delighted, and planned to drop by their house the next afternoon when Julian would be home from school.

Julian was a huge man. Well over six feet, he weighed 230 pounds. He was an athlete in college, but when he got his B.A. he dropped all sports and concentrated on obtaining higher degrees and on his present job as instructor in a small college. His body became fat and stiff.

"Julian, I'm sorry your back hurts," I said. "I'd like to show you something that might help. Why don't you get down on the floor."

"No."

"What?"

"I don't want to get down on the floor."

"Oh, Julian," his wife hissed, "for heaven's sake."

I could hear the ice in her voice. His face was flushed. Quickly I said that there was another exercise excellent for low back pain: it consisted of squatting.

"Hold on to something." I was about to say, "Hold on to the doorknob," but when I looked at his mass I said instead, "Why don't you hold onto the leg of the grand piano and slowly let yourself down. Down—down—down—like this." I demonstrated. "Feet apart, back straight, bend your knees, but don't lean forward. Hold on to the piano leg and lower yourself down very slowly—down—down. Your hips will automatically tuck under, and your back, now functioning with a curve in it, will be stretched and straightened."

He grunted his assent, walked to the piano, spread his feet apart, grasped the piano leg and started bending his knees. He did not lean forward but he was so stiff that he had to lean back. Down—did I see the piano moving? Down—good grief it *was* moving. Down—the piano had gained momentum and was rolling toward him. He had to let go and toppled over on the floor.

He was furious. He thrashed about and had a difficult time getting up. I had not realized that anyone, especially a young person, could be that stiff. He was humiliated and angry. I apologized profusely and left as soon as possible. This experience taught me several things:

1. Never, *never* offer advice unless the sufferer begs for it.

2. The Squat is an advanced exercise. Do not let anyone try it until he can Ride a Horse, Rock the Pelvis and do the Groucho Walk.

3. Make sure he knows how to get up off the floor before he tries it.

The Groucho Walk

Do you sometimes wake up in the morning with a terrific pain in your lower back? It goes away as the day progresses, but the first hour is sheer hell. Often you just stay in bed because it hurts so. If you are one of these, try the Groucho Walk.

Do you remember how Groucho Marx used to walk around, with his knees deeply bent? He looked so silly, puffing on his cigar, waving his eyebrows, with his knees sticking out in front of him.

I doubt if he knew he was doing a wonderful back exercise, but it does stretch those muscles of the lower back that can go into spasm during sleep. **(Fig. 31)**

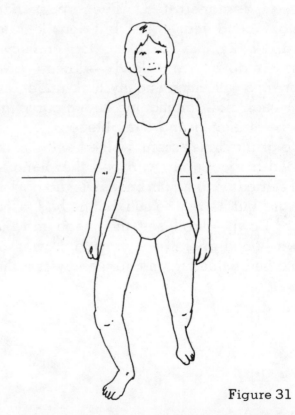

Figure 31

I once worked in a retirement home, and tried to interest the residents in a class in movement. I didn't get very far with that project. There was one resident who was particularly hostile. She said she could not imagine why the board of directors had hired me.

"Why did they hire an activities director?" she asked. "And why do you think you can teach us exercises? This house is like a club, an exclusive club. We will do what we please."

Recognizing defeat, I went to the door and started to bow myself out. "But I like you," she said. "I expect you to come and see me often." A few days later she was lying in wait for me in the hall. "Come to my room, I have to talk to you."

When we had privacy, she told me about her early morning backache. "Sometimes it's so bad I cannot get dressed and I have to go without breakfast."

I told her about the Groucho Walk and demonstrated it for her.

A few days later she walked all the way down to my office.

"I just had to tell you," she said. "The Groucho Walk has changed my life. I get out of bed doing it. It is like a miracle. It stretches out the pain right away. And the best thing about it is that I get laughing so much as I do it that I laugh out loud. It's marvelous to start the day laughing."

Transfer of Weight

This may seem really too simple to bother with, but it is extremely important, as you will see in a later chapter.

Stand with your feet at least a foot and a half or two feet apart. Let your knees be loose, not locked but not really bent.

Ride a Horse for a few minutes—let your hips be loose. Think about where your weight is, try to distribute it equally.

Now shift your weight so it is entirely on your left foot. Your right foot is still on the ground, as a balancer. Shift your weight to your right foot with your left foot balancing you.

Now bend the knee of the leg on which your weight rests. As your knee of that leg bends, the other knee automatically straightens, or will, if your feet are far enough apart. Shift your weight from side to side, slowly.

Remind yourself to do this any time you are standing, whether waiting for a bus, in line at a supermarket, or washing dishes. Simply shift your weight from one foot to the other.

Swinging

Swinging is simple—it's transferring your weight from side to side, and allowing your body to follow the motion freely.

Place your feet at least two and a half to three feet apart. Keep your knees loose—slightly bent. Start to sway slowly from side to side, transferring your weight from one foot to the other as you sway.

Then bend the knee on the side toward which you are swaying. Let your arms go with the motion so they swing out, swing out from side to side. **(Figs. 32a, b, c, and d)**

Keep your neck loose, too, so your head is swinging. Now let your body turn as you swing, with your arms following loosely so they wrap themselves around you. Don't try to do anything special with them, just release them from your body so they can move freely.

Be aware of how it feels to be loose. It's important not to go too fast because you don't want to get dizzy or exhausted. There really are no right or wrong ways to swing. What you want is to feel loose and happy.

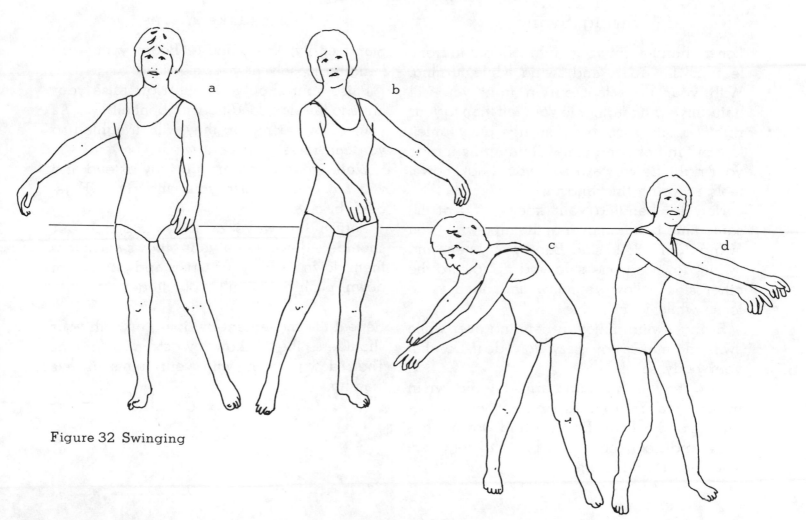

Figure 32 Swinging

Swing, Swing

For a change, put your right foot out in front, feet still far apart, and swing while turning. With your right foot out in front you will naturally swing farther to your left than to your right. So, after a couple of swings, put your left foot out in front and you will naturally turn to your right. Be very aware of your back, how it feels as you swing and turn.

Now try bending your knees, and at the same time bending over at the hips while you swing from side to side. Bend your knees and swing down on one side and up toward the other side. Allow your jaw and head to be loose while you do this.

Swing, swing. Enjoy. If bending over while swinging makes you dizzy, don't do it. Do what your body says!

Now let your head and arms hang down in front of you. Your knees are bent, your hands are near the floor. Bob up and down, your back and neck loose as a piece of seaweed. Your head bobbles gently.

Arms Like Waves

Stand easily, knees loose. Begin with arms hanging loosely at your sides.

Raise your shoulders first. Now raise your arms to the side, leading with bent elbows. As your elbows come up they will straighten so you can raise your bent wrists.

When your wrists are up they extend and you are able to raise your fingertips. (**Figs. 33a, b, c, and d**)

Return the wave as follows: push your shoulders down, bend your elbows and press them down, bend your wrists and push them down, push down with your fingertips.

Repeat the movement by going up with your shoulders, then elbows, wrists and fingers. Then down again, with your joints always leading.

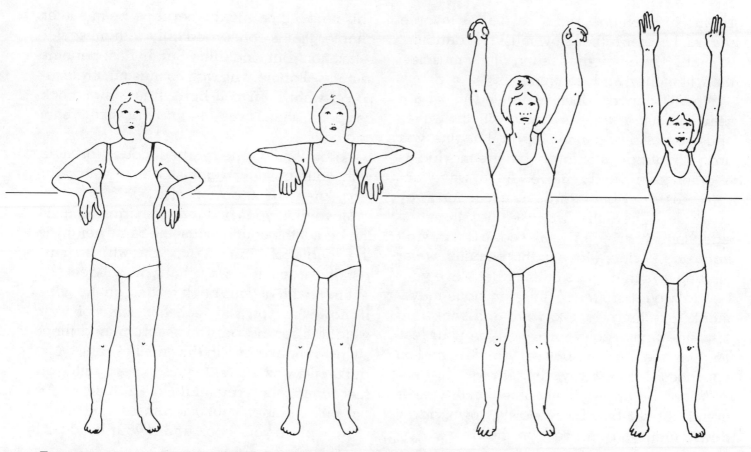

Figure 33 Arms Like Waves a   b   c   d

The Seaweed Dance

Let us turn on the radio or play a favorite record. I prefer rather slow music for dancing, so that I can enjoy the feeling of my muscles, their stretches and contractions.

When I dance, I like to pretend that I am seaweed in the ocean, swaying with the waves and the pulse of the sea. Try it. Imagine you are without bones or joints, but are moving as a giant kelp would move. As a wave approaches, sway backwards, as it recedes, sway forwards. When the water eddies from the side, feel your long seaweedness swaying from side to side. Move in this beautiful water all the ways that you can imagine. Move your feet as well, continuing this sensuous movement. Take long steps forward and backward and sideways. Feel your weight on your feet, on your heels, on the balls of your feet, and on your toes. Move, sway, dip, enjoy.

When you are tired, imagine that the tide is going out, far out. Sway slowly down, down, down, until you can rest on the floor.

The Super Rest

This next recipe should, perhaps, be in a later chapter that is concerned only with muscular relaxation. But since this Super Rest pertains to body alignment as well as muscular relaxation, I want to give it here. It is a swayback corrector, that I was taught over sixty years ago.

Lie on the floor near a bed, couch, or table with your buttocks against it and with your legs, knees bent, on top of it.

Move until your buttocks are firmly against the bed. If the couch is just the same height as the length of your thigh, you will be suspended in such a way that you will feel the entire length of your back resting on the floor. If, however, you still feel that some of your weight is resting on your sacrum, and there still is a slight curve in the small of your back, put a pillow or two under your knees, until you feel comfortable. You might like a small, rather flat pillow under your sacrum as well.

Now place your book under your head (as I

have suggested on page 52). Your shoulders are flat on the floor, your hands beside you. Once you are in this position, be aware that the bones in your back are resting heavily on the floor. Concentrate on them. Wiggle and adjust your position, until you can clearly feel each bone against the floor.

Now close your eyes, release your jaw, and say slowly to yourself, "My back is long. My shoulders are wide. My neck is long. My jaw and neck are free."

Breathe slowly. Repeat again and again,

"My back is long, my shoulders wide, my neck is long and my jaw and neck are free."

Say it slowly. The muscles that have been tight for so long will gradually loosen, and you will loosen, too. You may even drop off to sleep for a minute or two.

When you get up, I think you will feel refreshed and your back will feel long and straight.

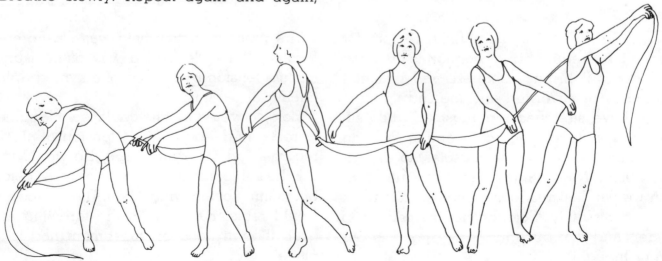

~ CHAPTER FOUR ~

Recipes For Loosening

Loosening is the essence of these recipes for comfort. Loosening brings comfort to the body that hurts. It brings calmness and peaceful feelings to the worried and the sad.

We have stretched our muscles while sitting, and while moving about, and in so doing we came to know those muscles, to experience them. Now that they have our full attention we can learn to loosen them and to relax them completely. Science has helped us to understand that our muscles respond to our every thought.

The pioneer in this field was Dr. Edmund Jacobson.[1] He devised a way of measuring muscle tension by the use of a kymograph, a tracing apparatus.

He discovered that he could teach a subject to relax so deeply that no tension at all was recorded on the kymograph. He would then ask the subject to remain as relaxed as before, but to think of throwing a ball. The kymograph would register tension in the throwing arm, even though no overt movement had taken place!

This experiment, performed in the 1920s, demonstrated the relationship between our thoughts and what happens in our bodies. The mere *thought of* something...elicits a physical response.

If we lie down to rest, but think of chores that need doing, we are not, in fact, resting, because our muscles are behaving, in a miniscule manner, as though we were actually doing those chores. Nothing has been accomplished, but we will still arise feeling tired.

Dr. Jacobson, as you can see, was the American grandfather of biofeedback. He applied his technique to the measurement of tension in the tongue. A trained subject would relax his tongue, so there was no tension demonstrable, then he would be asked to think in words, to talk to himself silently. Immediately the kymograph would register tension in the tongue.

A barricade, on the road to "thinking loose," is this habit that so many of us have of talking to ourselves. We make lists in our minds, lists of groceries to be bought, of duties to be done, or of conversations past or future.

This kind of constant mental activity is referred to in Asian literature as "the monkey mind." It skitters and jumps from thought to thought, but never is still. Quieting the mind is the aim of much meditative practice and is, say the sages, the beginning of wisdom.

You may be too frightened to allow your body to be loose. Many people feel more safe being tight than being relaxed.

One young woman, preparing for the birth of her first child, had a hard time believing and trusting in herself. But eventually, she found her loving center, by being completely loose and accepting. She found it to be pleasant, and so will you.

Please read this next section on relaxing into a tape recorder, if you have one. Read slowly so that when you play the tape back to yourself you can experience it fully so that your body will have time to accept your instructions.

If you do not have a tape recorder, read it aloud to yourself while you are comfortably lying down. Read it aloud several times, and eventually you will memorize it.

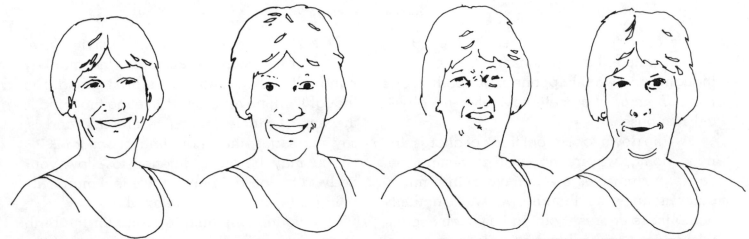

Figure 34 Face and Tongue

The first step toward quieting the mind is to relax the face and the tongue. This is a necessary preliminary for loosening the rest of our muscles.

Face and Tongue

Think of your entire face. (Fig. 34)

Make a grimace. Stick out your jaw, then pull it in. Make a fish face, then a big grin. Wiggle your nose. Wiggle your eyebrows and scalp. Do all the funny things you can think of with your face.

When your face, in general, feels that it has been moved all over, go to your tongue.

The tongue is composed of muscles. Therefore, as we can control muscles when we know them, let us learn to know the tongue.

Stick out your tongue as far as it will go. Pull it in, swallow. Stick it out and try to touch your chin. Bring it in, then try to touch your nose. Try to touch your right ear. Try to touch your left ear. Pull in your tongue, relax and swallow.

As you move your tongue through these exercises, be aware of the stretch on the roof of your mouth, and the tension underneath the

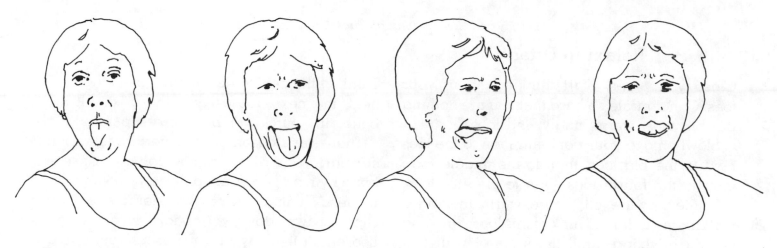

Figure 34 Face and Tongue

tongue when trying to touch your chin. Note the opposite sensations when reaching for your nose. A tiny muscle weaves from your tongue to a small bone below each ear. Feel the stretch in that muscle as your tongue reaches sideways.

Finally, stretch your whole body and give a nice big yawn. Now concentrate on the tip of your tongue until it starts to tingle. Think of nothing but the tip of your tongue and enjoy the tingling.

Then direct the tingling down to the base of your tongue. Think down your throat and loosen your vocal chords. Direct your atten-tion up the back of your throat, then to the roof of your mouth.

Let your whole mouth, throat and tongue, be so loose that you cannot think in words. Try to keep this concentration and enjoy the sensa-tion of utter silence.

You are speaking no words, which can be blissful. In fact, writing this section has taken days, for when I think about my tongue, it automatically gets so loose that I cannot think at all.

Now do you dare to experience being loose all over? The following exercise takes about six minutes.

Relaxing Utterly

Close your eyes. Start thinking about your toes. Concentrate so hard that you are nothing but big toes, warm, tingly and loose.

Slowly move your concentration to the toes next to the big toes, then to the middle toes, then to the fourth toes, then to the little toes. Imagine they are jelly, loose, warm, melting—melting in sunlight. Think of this loose, melting feeling traveling, until the soles of your feet are jelly, as are your insteps. The bones in your feet are melting also. Think of your heels and let them melt.

Direct the calves of your legs to be loose. Your shins are loose. The bones of your knees are loose. Let your thigh bone turn to jelly. Let all the muscles in your thighs be loose, loose. Let your buttocks relax. Let the lowest part of your spine, your coccyx, and all the tissues surrounding that area relax. Loosen your anus.

Then move your concentration slowly to your spine. Think of each bone becoming loose, and all the muscles falling away. Unhook one vertebra, so that it is just lying there.

Think of the next vertebra, unhook it, then the next, the next—loose—and the next. All the bones in your lower back are separated.

Then start loosening the vertebrae which support your ribs—loose—loose—loose—bone by bone, up your spine, to your shoulder blades. Think of your shoulder blades just slipping away down your back—loose—loose. Loosen all the way up the rest of your spine, way up to your neck.

Slip down to your fingers—let them be loose. Think about your thumbs, so that they begin to feel loose and tingly. Then think about the index finger on your left hand, then your middle finger, then the fourth finger, then the little finger. Feel them tingling, then think about your right hand—thumb, index finger, middle finger, fourth finger, little finger.

All your fingers are warm, tingling. Your palms are loose, warm. The backs of your hands are loose, warm. This looseness slides over your wrists, up the insides of your arms—loose—loose.

Loosen the insides of your upper arms and move around to your chest. Allow the looseness to slide up the backs of your forearms to your elbows. Let your elbows dissolve and then be loose in the backs of your upper arms.

Feel the looseness sliding around to your throat. Let your jaw drop. Let your tongue be loose. Release your nose. Unfocus your eyes, so they are so loose that you see nothing but gray. Think of this looseness, spreading to the top of your head, then flowing down, over and through you. Loose—loose—loose—just let go all over.

Slowly yawn and stretch. Please do not jump up and start running, as soon as the tape is finished. Lie there for a few minutes—allow yourself to wake up slowly. Think about how it feels to relax your muscles. Stretch—slowly come back to everyday business. As a matter of fact, if you just lie there perhaps you'll go to sleep. And why not?

There are other ways to achieve muscular relaxation. For example, there is the Jacobson method, tightening the muscles in one arm, then letting go and seeing how loose you can be in that arm before starting the same treatment in the other arm, then the legs, and so on. Or, imagine you can feel one leg becoming heavy and warm. When you feel that, try it on the other leg; then one arm, then the other arm. Or, imagine you are so heavy you are going to sink through the floor, or that you are so loose and light you float away.

Any of these will work, but I personally like my way, because emphasis is placed on the back, which supports us and is under constant tension. Also, I think it is good to relax the mouth and tongue, as well as the anus, so that our nourishing tube, the digestive tract, can be loose and open.

☙ CHAPTER FIVE ☙

Recipes for Imaginings

Whatever system you use for relaxation requires some imagination. I believe that the imagination needs stretching just as much as our muscles need stretching. I am going to give your some visualizations, and I hope they will start you on your journeys into unknown spaces.

When we were children we were told, "Stop daydreaming. Get on with your homework." Daydreams are really imaginings of our idealized world. We grew up aware that such dreams were not sanctioned by our elders, but now that we ourselves are elders we can approve, enjoy, and use our imaginations to our advantage.

When we were younger, working at raising a family or laboring in a store or office, we had days when we didn't feel like moving, but we had to. We drank quarts of coffee and somehow managed. Today, as elders, aren't we lucky? We can go back to bed and after a second rest usually feel like getting up.

Fatigue and hunger are causes of many depressions and unreasonable flares of anger. When we think about it, we have all experienced such anger, or have borne the brunt of it.

There is another kind of depression that is not healed by food or rest—the depression that is the *poor me* trap. I suppose we have all been in this trap at one time or another. We have all heard people who were caught in it saying: "No one has ever suffered as I have suffered. No one else has endured such misfortune. And now I am alone. What will become of me?"

Many of us who are old have lost our spouses and dear friends. We live on fixed incomes that are not sufficient for today's needs. And we do *not* know what will become of us. No one knows how life will end. If we spend our days concentrating on these dreary facts, how can we not be depressed? But I think we have a choice.

One choice could be that we can make ourselves even more depressed by our visualization of how bad things are, constantly enumerating them to ourselves. On the other hand, we can choose to imagine ourselves in joyous situations.

For instance, let us imagine we are on a beach. Sometimes I visualize a beach I know, a stretch of sand beside the sea. Picture your beach, wherever you are happy, and start running, running swiftly, run as you ran as a child, or would like to have been able to run. Run like the wind. Feel your feet in the sand. Feel your heel as it hits the sand and your toes as you spring forward. Feel the breeze in your face, smell the delicious salt of the sea. Is the sun in your eyes or is it behind you? Hear the sound of the waves and the cries of the gulls, and run, faster and faster until a magic thing happens and you find you don't have to touch the ground anymore. You can sail over rocks. You can sail to the top of a cliff and glide down the other side. You can run on the water and leap from wave to wave.

It is magic and it is happy—and you probably will run into a deep sleep. This is often very effective visualization to help you get to sleep at night, at those times when stretching and body movements are not enough.

Or... you can run through a meadow of flowers where a small brook meanders. Feel the grass on your feet. Smell the sweetness of the blossoms. Leap back and forth across the stream. A meadowlark sings in the crystal air. How lovely, how lovely.

Or...you can climb a mountain, walking steep narrow paths, clambering over rocks and then down into a deep ravine filled with the smell of moss and damp earth. You can climb up the other side, zigzag up and up, use all your strength to scramble upward.

You can translate this visualization into any kind of physical activity, any sport in which you excelled in your youth, or that you always wanted to try. Imagine yourself playing the perfect game. Imagine driving a ball down the fairway, across the bunker and onto the green. You execute the putt with ease for a hole in two. Or, play a tennis match with one of the world's experts whom you confound with your smashing serve, your agile footwork, your astonishing backhand. Or dance like Martha Graham, Margot Fonteyn, Mikhail Baryshnikov. You are limited only by your imagination.

This is not just a childish daydream, for in the imagining of this strenuous activity your muscles move, not much, but they are stimulated. I enjoy watching dance performances and always feel weary the next day as though I had had some very strenuous activity. And of course I have—for when I see Baryshnikov leap into the air, I leap with him although I do not move from my seat.

It is exciting to think of this kind of movement. The spirit soars with the body. It is a great improvement over feeling sorry for vanished youth.

Renewal

Another recipe for health and comfort is to go to the country or to a park. Take off your shoes, walk on the earth or the grass. When you are tired, sit under a tree, sense its energy—partake of it. Feel the earth beneath you—absorb its strength. Mary Sue Fitzgerald has expressed this well in her poem, "Renewal."[1]

The hike was long

At the top
she sank down
into the high grass.

The sky drew her eyes
closed them.

Her body flowed along the earth
deep into its crevices.

Roots grew
from thighs and calves
from back and shoulders
through the grass.

From outstretched arms
the fingers
softly
touched the ground
delicately found their way
into the rich soil.

Firmly held
she rose with the earth
to the horizon
together they slid down
into the sky
floating smoothly
into orbit.

She moved on earth's axis
felt the surge of its turning
swung with it
into night
into day.

Earth fluids came
gently flowing
into her body
renewing plasma.

Cells were re-born
divided
grew.

She lifted her body
in exultation
and moved again
into the world

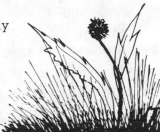

A Body Trip

There are times when we need less active, more intellectual or philosophical imaginings. Sometimes when I am feeling slightly ill, I like to take a trip through my body. When you feel tired and discouraged, take this trip with me.

Lie down, relax your tongue, and think about your body becoming looser and looser. Maybe you will want to play the tape you made.

Generally we don't think of our bodies at all, unless they hurt, and then we are angry because they do. Take this trip to marvel at the body's functioning and then visit the hurting part to comfort it.

To do this, pretend you are very small, so small that when you take a breath in, you can sail in with your breath to your lungs. You find that you are in an *alveolus,* one of the little air sacs that expand as you take a breath and become limp as you breathe out. It is breezy here, like being in a concertina, so hop a ride on a red corpuscle that has just taken on oxygen. Hang on tightly while you are being pumped through the left *atrium* and *ventricle* of your heart to the *aorta,* that great highway that carries oxygenated blood. You descend quickly, but slow down as arteries branch off and become smaller and smaller. Finally you find yourself in a capillary of your right foot. Here the oxygen your corpuscle picked up in your lung will hop off as you are going slowly through the capillary. The capillary is so small that the corpuscles must go in single file. You notice that the capillary itself is made of single cells placed side by side with slight spaces in between. These spaces allow the oxygen and nutrients in the blood to leave the vessel and make their way to a waiting cell. You watch what is happening around the corpuscle and are amazed at how watery it is outside the capillary. Each individual cell is bathed in fluid in which the nutrients and the oxygen molecules float to a cell, where they pass directly through the cell wall. At the same time, carbon dioxide and garbage are pushed out of the cell to float around in the fluid (just like throwing the garbage into a canal). They slip through a space in the capillary where the carbon dioxide pulls itself aboard a red corpuscle. Your distaste at seeing garbage in the fluid is relieved when you become aware that the garbage never re-enters another cell, but enters only into a blood vessel.

You are so involved in the activity of the life around you that you realize you are scarcely moving. You remember that there is no pump in your toes to pump you upward, so you feel a little nervous until you see that the tiny tunnel through which you have been moving is itself moving up and down. As you begin to pick up speed, you reach a larger vein and go still faster. Finally you are whizzing upward through the *interior vena cave* (the largest vein) and are dumped into the right atrium of your heart. Then you are pumped to the right ventricle, which pumps you again to the lung. The whole trip has only taken about twenty-three seconds!

You are quite breathless from the last moments of rapid travel, but before you can decide to jump off when the carbon dioxide leaves your corpuscle, new oxygen has joined you and you are zipped through the heart again and are started downward. Soon you slow down as you enter a small *arteriole* and then you are in another capillary where all the cells surrounding it are moving up and down. You feel you must be in some dough that is being kneaded. Then you realize that you are traversing the lining of your stomach, which is, indeed, kneading the food you have recently eaten, mixing it with pepsin and hydrochloric acid, breaking it down until it becomes *chyme,* a liquid that pours from your stomach through the *pyloris* into the intestine, gathering other juices as it goes.

Of course, you return to your heart and thence to your lungs again, to be rid of the carbon dioxide and to pick up more oxygen.

On your next trip you might visit your small intestine, that marvelous tube that averages twenty-three feet in length and one inch in diameter and that is packed neatly into the abdominal cavity. In the small intestine the nutrients that have been extracted from your food are absorbed into your bloodstream by means of an astonishingly clever design. The tube is not like a garden hose with a straight interior. No, in order to make more space for absorption, the lining, or *mucosa,* is folded back and forth in tiny pleats which are covered with *villi,* minuscule fingerlike projections barely visible to the naked eye. *Villi* are packed so closely together that the interior of the intestine appears lined with velvet. *Villi* move constantly, pushing the chyme along. Each *villus* contains a blood vessel and a lymph vessel, which gather the nutrients into your bloodstream. Now, imagine you are inside a *villus* and are watching nutrients come aboard. Isn't it amazing? Isn't it astonishing? Have you ever thought, in intricate detail, how the food you eat reaches your muscles, so you have the strength to move? You cannot help but be proud of your intestines when you think about them.

I am aware that these imaginary excursions into body intricacies are highly simplified. They may seem unimportant, but I want you to appreciate the wonders within you. Love and respect these things that go right, then with your imagination go into the place or system that is causing you pain. For example, it is a great help to imagine that your arthritic arm or leg or joint is a baby. When a baby cries, you comfort it. You hold it in your arms and say, "There, there, it's all right. You are all right. Let go, let go."

There are many times when this will help you, when you will feel your tissues loosening, letting go. The sensation of discomfort may still be with you, but it no longer will be frightening. You will—and can—cope with it. And, as you now are aware of the effectiveness and the marvel of your body, you will be surprised at how much more confidence you have in yourself.

A Visit to a Cell

Another imagining I find exhilarating is to pay a visit to a cell. Lewis Thomas writes in his marvelous book, *The Lives of a Cell,*[2] that a cell is like the earth in its complexity. From reading his book I have dreamed up a place that I visit in my imagination. I like to go there when I am feeling, not ill, but not energetic and a little lonely. So come with me, if you will, on a fantasy.

First we become small, smaller even than when we took a trip through the body, for to enter a cell we must be able to slip through one of the pathways in a capillary, then swim in the canal of fluid that surrounds the cell and enter into the cell through an opening in its membrane. We are lucky to get in. The cell is selective as to what shall enter, but we have received special dispensation for this visit.

The membrane encloses a space that seems enormous, as it needs to be to encompass so many activities. In the center is the nucleus, round in shape with transparent walls. We are not free to enter the nucleus. It is busy coiling its chromosomes, which carry its genetic information, but we are free to wander around in the *cytoplasm.* This watery substance is filled with all kinds of machines and animals, for, it turns out, there are tiny organelles such as *ribosomes,* rounded bodies that play an important part in the manufacture of protein molecules. There is also the *endoplasmic reticulum,* constructed of delicate membranes so interconnected as to form a network of tiny canals, with *ribosomes* covering the whole. Communicating with this is the *Golgi apparatus,* an array of parallel membranes arranged as flattened sacs. It is believed that this apparatus is concerned with the export of substances produced by the *endoplasmic reticulum.* It seems as though the endoplasmic reticulum is a manufacturing plant and the *Golgi* is the packaging and shipping division and both are made of living membrane.

Then there are other organelles called *lysosomes,* tiny closed sacs containing powerful digestive enzymes that are capable of breaking down worn-out parts of the cell itself as well as other substances that may have entered the cell.

My favorite creatures in this strange place are the *mitochondria,* the energy producers within us. Lewis Thomas says of them:

At the interior of our cells, driving them, providing the oxidative energy that sends us out for the improvement of each shining day, are the mitochondria, and in a strict sense they are not ours. They turn out to be little separate creatures, the colonial posterity of migrant prokaryocytes, probably primitive bacteria that swam into ancestral precursors of our eukaryotic cells and stayed there. Ever since, they have maintained themselves and their ways, replicating in their own fashion, privately, with their own DNA and RNA quite different from ours. They are as much symbionts as the rhizobial bacteria in the roots of beans. Without them, we would not move a muscle, drum a finger, think a thought.[3]

I like to hang around these mitochondria. I'd love to talk with them, but they are too busy to bother with me. Thomas says:

My centrioles, basal bodies, and probably a good many other more obscure tiny beings at work inside my cells, each with its own special genome, are as foreign, and as essential, as aphids in anthills. . . . . I like to think that they work in my interest, that each breath they draw for me, but perhaps it is they who walk through the local park in the early morning, sensing my senses, listening to my music, thinking my thoughts.[4]

This journey makes me feel very close to the other creatures of the earth. For all of them, from whales to mosquitoes, mitochondria are busy.

How can I feel lonely when billions of cells are doing so much for me, and for you, and for all living creatures? My visit to a cell makes me realize that the earth is one enormous cell and you and I are workers in it. We are very much connected.

Another trip I like to take is to enter into an atom. The smallness needed to accomplish this feat is beyond my imagining, so I don't try to do that. I simply find myself in an atom.

Here the space is immense, there is no crowding, there is movement, and the silence dissolves into an echo, or a memory, of music, of mighty chords and harmonies, resolving and dissolving. I float and watch the atomic particles move in their stately dance. Of course I know that from the view point of the world, the movement of atomic particles is swift and whirling, but when I am smaller than an atomic particle, my experience is one of slowness. Bits or waves of energy break off to dance their own dance, change into something else, and dance away to combine with other particles in other atoms. The movement is playful and happy. I feel that I am at the core of the universe and can experience all things. The discovery of Fritjof Capra's description of his experience was therefore an event of deep meaning to me:

> I was sitting by the ocean one late summer afternoon, watching the waves rolling in and feeling the rhythm of my breathing, when I suddenly became aware of my whole environment as being engaged in a gigantic cosmic dance. Being a physicist, I knew that the sand, rocks, water and air around me were made of vibrating molecules and atoms, and that these consisted of particles which interacted with one another by creating and destroying other particles. I knew also that the Earth's atmosphere was continually bombarded by showers of "cosmic rays," particles of high energy undergoing multiple collisions as they penetrated the air. All this was familiar to me from my research in high-energy physics, but until that moment I had only experienced it through graphs, diagrams and mathematical theories. As I sat on that beach my former experiences came to life; I "saw" cascades of energy coming down from outer space, in which particles were created and destroyed in rhythmic pulses; I "saw" the atoms of the elements and those of my body participating in this cosmic dance of energy; I felt its rhythm and I "heard" its sound, and at that moment I *knew* that this was the Dance of Shiva, the Lord of Dancers worshipped by the Hindus.[5]

❧ CHAPTER SIX ❧

Recipes for Walking

Doctors tell us that no matter what kind of exercise we do, we also need to walk. Walking seems to be the ideal way to keep the circulatory system in good shape. The body is accustomed to walking. We, the human species, walked for millions of years before we learned to ride. The rhythm of walking is part of our being, just as the rhythm of waves is part of the sea.

Such considerations, however, are not what influence the medical profession, for they know that walking helps the heart to pump and the blood to move. Any kind of movement increases the gusto with which the blood moves through the body and walking is an activity that can be sustained over a long period of time.

We need not run nor jog, we just have to find our correct rhythm. We need to stimulate our hearts, so the rate of beating increases by a small amount, and we need to sustain that increase over a period of time. The correct amount of increase in heart rate is an individual matter—something that you should discuss with your doctor.

The increase in crime on city streets has terrified many people and has made them prisoners in their own homes, shut-ins crippled by fear. Walking is a less simple pleasure than it used to be.

I talked recently with Joel Kirsch,[1] teacher of self-protection without violence. One concept of his teaching is that the victim invites violence. You will probably say, "What utter nonsense. No one wants to be mugged. Why would anyone invite it?" Of course no one wants to be mugged—*but*—more muggings seem to occur to people who walk in a certain way than they do to people who walk in another fashion. So, isn't it worthwhile to examine the walk and posture of those whom muggers call "easy hits"?

Joel gave me an article by Betty Grayson and Morris I. Stein called, "Attracting Assault: Victims' Nonverbal Clues."[2] This report points out quite clearly that differences between postural and gestural movement can make the difference between being mugged or not. Apparently, this group of prison inmates was asked to review videotapes of people walking in high assault areas of New York City. The tapes were than analyzed by movement specialists who used Labanalysis, an established system of movement notation for the study of nonverbal communication. Both methods reached the same conclusion. The following is a summary from their excellent report:

> As the taped sequences were presented to this group, the prisoners were asked to talk about the videotaped persons in terms of their being targets for assault. These evaluations, determined by the prisoners and in their own language, were used to establish a rating scale from 1 to 10. The same scale was used later by a second set of prisoners, 53 inmates also convicted of assaultive crimes, to rate the tapes on the individuals' assault potential....
>
> The major difference between victim and non-victim as perceived by criminal respondents and as described by the Labanalysis notation seems to be the difference that exists between postural and gestural movement.
>
> The terms posture and gesture refer to how much of the body participates in a movement. In postural movement, the initiation of the movement comes from the body center, while gestural movement is initiated from the body's periphery.[2]

Postural movement is when everything works together. Gestural movement is when hands and feet move in an unconnected fashion, and the result is awkward, unbalanced.

The authors of this report concluded that the greatest statistical difference in movement between victim and non-victim is in the walk. The greatest number of victims walked with the lopsided, unilateral walk—right leg and right arm forward at the same time, left leg and left arm forward at the same time. Non-victims used the easy contralateral walk—right arm forward as the left leg swings forward, the left arm accompanies the right leg.

Walk around the room right now and see which movement is natural for you. If you are a unilateral walker—right leg with right arm—please turn to the description of Crawling in the chapter for Movers, page 63. As we said, there seems to be a relationship between crawling and some kinds of body difficulties. If you want to change to being a contralateral walker, crawling will help you.

> The prime difference between perceived victim and non-victim groups, . . .seems to revolve around a "wholeness" or consistency of movement. Non-victims have an organized quality about their body movements, and they function comfortably within the context of their own bodies. In contrast, the gestural movement of victims seems to communicate inconsistency and dissonance.[3]

Twenty years ago, in an article whose source has been forgotten, there was another point that has bearing on this subject. It was written by a reformed pick-pocket, who said that all pick-pockets know that there are some people who cannot be robbed. His description of such people was that they are enveloped in angels' wings and cannot be touched.

I wish I knew exactly what he meant. A habit that has been with me for many years, and perhaps stemmed from that article, is that whenever I start my car I say, "Thank you for your protection." I don't know to whom I'm talking, certainly not a person, an entity perhaps, but I feel protected. We need all the help we can get, everywhere. It may help you to feel better when you give thanks for your protection. Try it before you walk.

No matter how much protection you have, use your body so that it utilizes the energy of the earth to hold you up and be part of the joyousness of life.

Find a friend, or friends, to walk with you. More muggings happen to single victims. Make friends with someone who lives near you and enjoy walking together. More about friends in the chapter, "Friends Are a Comfort."

"I would like to walk, but my feet hurt." I sympathize because I used to have a dreadful time finding something I could put on my feet that didn't make them hurt. I finally learned that pretty shoes with thin leather soles are not for me. I need crepe or composition soles with a bounce. As we get older the pads of fat on the soles of our feet diminish. A thick but lightweight sole is a help. Our feet may need more width to expand in, or possibly more length. We no longer need to be the Cinderella princess with tiny feet.

One of the greatest joys of being an elder is that we no longer need to follow fashions. That does not mean that we will be without style, for now we can have our own style that suits us and is comfortable. Talk to your friends, go hunting for shoes that are correct for you and be comfortable.

Remember when you are walking to try to use your feet properly. Make sure that both feet are pointing straight ahead, that you are not throwing one foot out to the side. Such crookedness can throw your weight off and be hard on your knees and your heels.

It might be a good idea while you are sitting here reading to practice the Sitting Duck Walk. Remember? Heel, ball, toe—heel, ball, toe, and then fast: heelballtoe, heelballtoe, heelballtoe. Now, stand up and practice the same thing as you walk around your room. Go slowly at first, heel, ball, toe; other foot: heel, ball, toe. Balance yourself with your hand against the wall, go slowly and think of each movement, each part of your foot, as it hits the floor. Now speed it up so you are walking at a normal rate, but try to keep your concentration on heelballtoe, heelballtoe.

Once you are outside you will have other things to think about but if your feet begin to hurt, heelballtoe it for a few minutes and see if they feel better.

The third objection that some people make to walking is that they say walking is boring. I find this hard to believe. If you leave your house carrying your same old boring thoughts and worries that you have been having all day you will have no time nor space in your head to see something new, think new thoughts, get new ideas. To enjoy your walk you must leave your worries and troubles at home. They will still be there when you return, if you really want them to be. The only thing you should take with you is what Wuji calls "the spark of life which weaves the tissues of your body."⁴ *That* is what you should walk with. Your tongue is loose so you are not talking to yourself, not having the same old arguments about the same old things. Your tongue is loose so your mind is open, ready to perceive more.

In the city you have buildings to see. Look at the details around windows and doors. Try to guess the age of the buildings, who lives there, what the inhabitants are like. Be aware of the people you pass, try to sense what they are feeling. Look at the outlines of the skyline. Look for growing things. Enjoy the trees that grow for your pleasure. If there is no sign of any growing thing, look for cracks in the pavement; sometimes, after a rain, moss will grow there. Of the richest and most beautiful green, this moss can be your garden.

If you are lucky enough to live in the country, each walk can be an ecstatic experience. Each blade of grass, each tree, bush and bird can be a delight but only if you can really see and hear. That again means a relaxed tongue and complete attention to NOW. I find it painful to walk with someone who talks but does not look, or rather does not see.

It may add to the interest of your walk, if you live in the city, to go to your local Historical Society and read about what happened on the very streets you are now treading. You may become intrigued with finding clues about buildings. Sidewalks or sewer covers are clues to antiquities.

If you are a country walker you can always study the botany of the plants you pass, or watch the birds and become a birder. There is no end of interesting things if you search for them. If you are fortunate enough to live by the sea, as I do right now, you can wake up very early and walk on the beach when there is a minus tide. This morning, where the beach is usually twenty to thirty feet wide, it was two hundred feet wide, wet and shining in the early sunlight.

Before you start walking remember the movements in this book. Stand with your feet planted solidly on the earth. Make sure that your knees are loose and your hips are loose and tucked under. Let the muscles of your back carry you upward. Let your neck be free so your head is able to go up and forward. Remember it is the crown of your head that is reaching for the stars. Let your shoulders be loose, not hunched up around your ears. Let your eyes be loose: soft eyes, unfocused, so that you have increased peripheral vision. Then before you go outside practice the Duck Walk: heelballtoe, heelballtoe.

Suddenly you will indeed feel that you are collected and centered. Walk with joy. You will not be molested. As Wuji says further, "Find, [be] aware and experience the spark of Life that weaves the tissues of your Body and Be with it. It is the only reality your Body has."[5] Feel this spark and walk with joy.

~ CHAPTER SEVEN ~

Friends Are A Comfort

Any book containing Recipes for Comfort would be incomplete if it did not talk about friends, for it seems obvious that friends are as comforting as moving our bodies, flexing our joints, stretching and relaxing our muscles. And, curiously enough, relaxing our bodies, which we have learned to do through stretching, has a lot to do with the quality of our friendships.

Happiness is having a friend who listens. Such a friend does not try to out-guess you and finish your sentence for you. A friend who listens does not give you advice unless you plead for it. A true friend will listen, and listen, and listen until you have talked your problem out and come to your own conclusion.

Such listening is rare. In our mechanized culture some people seem to have a notion that there is an answer to every question and that it behooves them to give an answer whether they understand our question or not. Have you ever had the experience of making a comment and receiving a long lecture about things you already know that had nothing to do with your comment?

A friend of mine said, "I have the sensation that no one hears me. It is as though I were talking to myself." Have you ever felt like that?

This longing to be heard was expressed beautifully by a woman who was working with many other women in a senior center, making gifts for an annual bazaar. She had a piquant face and often made wry comments in broken English that made others laugh. As she did so there was a half smile on her lips but her eyes were not merry. I was standing near her once, when she made such a sally, and noticed that after the laughter she sighed. There was a vacant chair next to her. I slipped into it.

"What's the matter?" I asked. "Why do you sigh so?"

She quoted something in Russian and then with an expansive gesture she said, "I long for someone to whom I can speak from the heart."

I know what she means. I think we all know what she means. True happiness is having a friend...who listens.

To find such a friend, we ourselves must first be good listeners and of course this means that we will be interested in the speaker and give her our complete attention. We will keep our tongues loose, not composing an answer in our heads while she is speaking. In that way we will really hear her and will be able to respond to her honestly. We will not start talking about something else, until we have exhausted the subject of her choice.

We also know that we invite confidences when our bodies are loose and free. The person who sits or stands with tight muscles is not encouraging friendship. Clenched jaws, crossed arms, tight raised shoulders, tight buttocks, stomach pulled in tightly with the resultant tight lower back, are giving signals that say, "stay away from me," even though the person making the signals is suffering from loneliness and is craving friends.

To illustrate, let me tell you of a time I worked part time for a doctor in a hospital. The man was pleasant at first but then became complaining and picky. I could do nothing right. He was so unpleasant that I decided to leave. Surely I could find another way to earn the small stipend that I was being paid.

The morning after I made this decision I was able to stop being defensive. When he began to pick on me, I could allow myself to relax, to let the muscles of my jaw and tongue be loose. I consciously relaxed the muscles of my belly and buttocks. Then I really heard him. I heard a man in pain. His hitting out at me was an attempt to rid himself of some of his pain.

"What's the matter?" I asked.

Suddenly I was deluged with his problems. He had been up all night with his sick children. His wife was also sick because she was so exhausted. She needed to go to Hawaii for a rest but there was no one to take care of the children. He was in the throes of being a young father with young children and a young wife. He needed someone to tell his troubles to. I stayed with him for several years. He never picked on me again.

When I could let go of my defences and of my concern over the job, a new and good relationship was established. The moral of the experience was, for me, "Don't hang on. Be loose. Let go." Our culture has conditioned us to be afraid of the new and unknown. As we are now in an age of change, we shall be wise to condition ourselves to meet what comes with equanimity.

We shall have the problem of where we are to meet potential friends. By what magic do we find them?

At one time we found our friends among our neighbors, and, indeed, up to about one hundred and fifty years ago, we, the elders (if we lived so long), lived on a farm with our children and grandchildren. We still worked, not the heavy work we did when we were young, but there was plenty to do. We worked until we died. Did we have this yearning then for friendship? Or were we too busy? Or did we find our hearts' communication with our children and grandchildren?

Our lives are so different today. We need to explore all the possibilities for enlarging our circle of acquaintances, from which we may find new friends.

Perhaps, after you have tried all the exercises in this book, you will want to find and join a class in movement. Moving with other people is pleasurable, for there you are all engaged in activities on a sub-verbal level. This can be a good basis for friendship, a sharing of an awareness of what the body is doing.

Fortunately, the importance of movement for the older adult (as well as for younger people), is becoming more and more recognized. Classes in body awareness, movement, yoga, aerobics, dance, swimming and T'ai Chi Ch'uan are being offered by Community Colleges, Adult Education Departments, Senior Centers, YWCA's and YMCA's, as well as by private studios.

Telephone around, find out what is available, then go visiting to decide what will be right for you. I made the mistake of joining a belly dance class the YWCA was presenting at a school near my home. I was in my sixties at the time and, as I was much more supple than many other women my age, it did not occur to me to use caution. During the first class of the series I kept up with the others, feeling mighty pleased with myself. But, alas, I had to spend the next two days in bed, with my body screaming at me for having been such an idiot. During the classes that followed I tried every new movement twice. The rest of the time I rested and admired the undulations of the teacher and her teenage students.

On the other hand, T'ai Chi Ch'uan, sometimes called "Chinese Shadow Boxing," was a delight to learn and is a delight to practice. It consists of 108 slow movements that my first teacher, Dr. Wong Lew, told me use every muscle in the body. "T'ai Chi is not for the impatient," he said, "for it takes a long time to learn and is done very slowly." Most instructors begin with a few basic movements, so do not be afraid that you might be asked to learn all of the movements at once.

Dr. Lew died fifteen years ago, but I still see some of the friends I made in that class. Some teachers will not teach T'ai Chi to anyone under forty, but T'ai Chi Master Al Chung-Liang Huang is a young man who also is a dancer, artist and philosopher. His seminars are a celebration of movement and dance, very different from traditional training, but exciting and joyous. If you can find a class in T'ai Chi in your area, why not investigate it?

Once you have found a few people you like, you might consider starting a class of your own, not as teacher but as organizer/expediter. Using this book as your guide, members could take turns leading the group. Move slowly and thoughtfully. After class you may want to have lunch together. I know of several groups of women who started working with me and then went on by themselves for years. Moving in your own way with your friends is a way to meet two of your greatest needs: movement and love.

Another great place to meet people is in adult education classes. A subject that fascinates you will attract others with the same interest and a common interest is a good basis for a friendship. There are classes in a great variety of subjects. Do not be intimidated if you have little education or experience in the subject of your choice. Plunge in and see what happens.

The writing of this book began some years ago when I saw an advertisement for "Autobiography, Writing from Experience," to be presented by the Emeritus College of the College of Marin. For years I had wanted to tell others about my work with the body, but I was convinced that I could not write. Perhaps this class could help me. The teacher showed me that it could.

There are adult education classes in almost anything you can think of: painting, sculpture, investments, literature, poetry, archeology, sewing or philosophy. Call your Department of Education and find out what is offered and where it is. And DON'T be afraid to start. It is a well known fact that no one knows everything.

If you have not been to a Senior Center because you didn't like the name or the idea, loosen up a bit, let go of your prejudices, and try one. If you don't like that one, try another. Most centers have classes of various sorts, from crafts and woodworking to sophisticated discussion groups. Counseling on health, housing and emotional problems is also available. Shop around. Many centers serve a hot lunch, good and nutritious at low cost, where you can eat with others in friendship. Look about you, the friend you are searching for may be there. Your church can also be an excellent source of new friendships. Many helping organizations depend on volunteers and would welcome you. You may find your friends there.

Groups are being formed all over the country to give support and help to those suffering from a chronic ailment. I go to a monthly "Better Breathers' Club," sponsored by the American Lung Association, to learn techniques that assist my chronically troubled lungs. The Arthritis Association is forming groups in many communities to help sufferers cope with their illness. Lupus sufferers have banded together and meet in many localities to give information and support to victims and their families. The Heart Association, the Cancer Association and many more are providing helping hands where friends may be found. Ask your doctor about such organizations.

Speaking of doctors, it would be a help to both you and your physician if you could think of him as a friend rather than as an adversary. My sister was so afraid of doctors that when she went to see one, she was unable to tell him why she was there. When she finally learned to write a list and read from it, she was too frightened to remember his answers. I've known other people with the same problems. It seemed to be a fear engendered in childhood and kept alive by the attitudes of an old-fashioned doctor. I knew a doctor who was trained before World War I who told me that he was taught not to tell his patients anything because if the patients thought he was God they would have more confidence in him. In that era it was also considered indelicate for women patients to ask personal questions.

The doctor cannot help us unless he knows exactly how and where we hurt. We can observe ourselves and take notes so that we will be able to give an accurate description of our symptoms. When he answers our questions in medical terms we can ask that he write them down in laymen's terms. Then you can write what you understood him to say and ask if you have heard correctly. This may annoy him at first, but eventually he will realize that you save him time by being precise and accurate in your questions and responses.

I would like to end this chapter by telling you of what seems to me to be an extraordinary happening in Italy. In 1951 an Italian psychiatrist, Dr. Antoinetta Bernardoni, founded a neighborhood support group known as "Popular Therapeutic Activity:"

> ...a new form of popular social and psychological process designed to help people integrate social realities with individual needs and to prevent the distortion of identity that occurs when that process of integration breaks down.... Its goal is to help people gain control over their own lives through an understanding and practice of community/neighborhood support.... Its theoretical base—the notion that personality development is inextricably tied to social contacts—has far-reaching implications for the treatment of mental illness as well.[1]

The "Activity," as it is known, meets twice a week:

> ...40 to 60 people meet in a local high school in Medina, Italy...ages [of the people are from] 5 to 85 years with the largest group represented in the 25 to 45 year range.... The members who share in this activity include farmworkers, school children, businessmen, housewives, teachers, cooperative leaders, artists, social workers, university students, factory workers, shopkeepers and farmers.... The atmosphere is warm and relaxed.
>
> Chairs are arranged in a circle and an individual with a need to speak begins to tell the others in the group about the problem she or he is having. Issues may include relations with husbands, wives, lovers, children, mothers, fathers, brothers, sisters, as well as relations with others in the neighborhood and at work....
>
> In the meetings all that is said is spoken to the whole assembly, not to one individual alone and friendship and mutual support are given freely, not purchased or sold....
>
> People discuss their problems with great candor, and a seeming lack of concern about confidentiality, and yet there is an unspoken understanding that there is a risk in personal revelation.

After an individual has described a painful situation, people begin to make suggestions. Perhaps someone will talk about being involved in a conflict similar to the one described and tell how she or he felt about the difficulty and what was most helpful in resolving it....

A frequent request is "Tell us what we can do that will be helpful to you." People are aided in solving their own conflicts and they are given the confidence to do this through receiving the support of so many concerned people....

The members agree that they do not want to be exploited or to exploit others. Those people who tend to be oppressive and authoritarian, do not find the meetings interesting for long, unless they seriously decide to change their mode of behavior. People looking for genuine transformation do not become bored because of the varied discussions, the multiplicity of issues which make the meetings interesting as well as challenging.... They are attentive in the meetings because they are learning a new way to live their lives, not engaged in a technique for "fixing" things....

There are no leaders because Popular Therapeutic Activity members recognize that too often leaders lead in ways that are not democratic and people follow in ways which increase opportunities for exploitation and stifle independence and self-help. [Dr. Bernardoni never comes to meetings for that reason.]...

[The meetings are all] free. Mutual help cannot be sold, but must be given. Part of the program's strength is derived from the opposition to marketing human assistance.[2]

I was so touched when I read this article that I wanted to add all of it to this chapter, but 16 pages are too much.

Wouldn't it be wonderful to belong to such a group, where all of us could speak from the heart and be heard?

CHAPTER EIGHT

How to Remember These Recipes for Comfort

When you read something in a book about movement, your head hears what the words say but your muscles do not. Your muscles have not been conditioned to move, so they need assistance in remembering. People who have been in my classes know these exercises, because I have taught the same movements over and over until their muscles, as well as their heads, remembered.

The movements I have presented here are few and basic. If you keep the image of a "stretching cat" in mind it will help you. Do not worry whether you are doing these movements exactly correctly. If you move slowly and gently, and it feels good, you are doing the right thing.

The important rule in all these movements, and, therefore, in remembering them, is to *pay complete attention to each second as it happens.*

In this work, as we have said before, this kind of attention has little to do with thinking about or trying to recall what you are to do next. Rather, it is focusing your attention on your body and receiving the messages it is sending you. For example, in doing the Sitting Twist, the simple movement where you pull yourself around to one side until you can go no farther, you will have found that by stopping and focusing on that spot and breathing into it, you are able to twist a little farther without forcing. It also helps to talk out loud while you move. This gives your muscles double instructions.

Let us go through a day together and figure out times and ways you can incorporate these movements into your daily living.

When you get out of bed in the morning and your back hurts, what do you do? You say, "I'm Groucho," and do the Groucho Walk, and laugh. You can't forget that. It is too simple and too silly to forget.

If your jaw or teeth hurt, open your mouth and stretch your tongue and your jaw. Sometimes we are so tense we clench or grind our teeth all night.

I like to move slowly and gently first thing in the morning, so I Ride a Horse as I brush my teeth. And I like to massage my feet while I loll in the bathtub. This tender treatment insinuates me slowly into the rest of the day.

You may be a morning person, and want to get going first thing when you wake up. So lie down on the floor with your book, on which you place your head, and say: "I am doing the Low Back Pain Remover. My head is raised slightly, slowly I bring my knees to my chest. I allow my lower back to stretch and straighten."

Then put your feet flat on the floor, with your knees bent, and say: "I am doing the Bridge. I raise my buttocks off the floor and come down bone, by bone, by bone, by bone, loosening my lower back, letting it roll like a bolt of silk upon the floor."

You then slide your arms above your head and say: "I am freeing the muscles of my arms, chest and shoulders while I do the Bridge." And do the Bridge again.

Now do a partial sit-up with your hands under the back of your head and say: "My arms are holding my head, allowing my neck muscles to be loose. I am lengthening my neck while I slowly lay my head tenderly upon a book. My neck is long and free."

Then you might say: "I am doing a Spiral Twist and stretch. My knees are bent, my feet flat on the floor. I put my right knee over my left bent knee and gently stretch to the right. Then I put my left knee over my right bent knee and gently stretch to the left. The spiral movement feels good. My back is supple. I move easily."

Of course, you will find your own words to describe what you are doing. But now that you are on the floor, you will need to get up, so first get on your hands and knees. As long as you are there you might as well arch your back like an Angry Cat and wag your tail like a Happy Puppy—another way to rock your pelvis and stretch your back. And now if you have room you can crawl. See how easy it is to remember?

If you are not a morning person you can do these stretches in the afternoon or at night. I like to do them before going to bed. They help me sleep.

Let us say now that the day has started and we leave our homes. It is surprising how much of the time we have to stand every day. We tend to stand as we wait for someone, or while we wait for a bus, or for our turn in a check-out line in a supermarket. Sometimes, after a long wait, we may feel as though we are going to collapse from so much standing. Indeed, we know that soldiers on parade sometimes faint when forced to stand at attention for too long. When we get tired from standing our bodies are saying to us, "DON'T JUST STAND THERE. MOVE!"

The following paragraphs explain what happens when we stand still.

Because of hydrostatic pressure, the venous pressure in the feet would always be about +90 mm. Hg in a standing adult were it not for the valves in the veins.... Every time one moves his legs he tightens his muscles and compresses the veins either in the muscles or adjacent to them, and this squeezes the blood out of the veins.... The valves in the veins...are arranged so that the direction of blood flow can be only toward the heart. Consequently, every time a person moves his legs or even tenses his muscles, a certain amount of blood is propelled toward the heart, and the pressure in the dependent veins of the body is lowered. This pumping system is known as the "venous pump"...it is efficient enough that...the venous pressure in the feet of a walking adult remains less than 25 mm. Hg.

If the human being stands perfectly still, the venous pump does not work, and the venous pressures in the lower part of the leg can rise to the full hydrostatic value of 90 mm. Hg in about 30 seconds....The pressures within the capillaries also increase greatly, and fluid leaks from the circulatory system into the tissue spaces....The legs swell, and the blood volume diminishes....As much as 15 to 20 percent of the blood volume is frequently lost from the circulatory system within the first 15 minutes of standing absolutely still.[1]

Because we do not have a heart pumping in each foot, we must keep moving. Do you remember the shifting weight movement? Simply shift your weight from the right foot to the left foot and back again.

If you have to stand in line for a very long time you may feel that you need to do more in order to keep the blood moving. Try standing on the right foot while you tip up your left heel, then lower that heel, shift your weight to the left and raise your right heel. It can be done slowly and inconspicuously. No one will notice and you will be saving yourself energy as well as preventing varicose veins as you wait.

This advice is different from what we were told as children. Remember? "Stand up straight and stand STILL." Children know that it is unnatural to stand still. We think they over-do their jiggling and bouncing and jumping, but we must learn from them. They know that *movement is life.*

When we are at home, we can do our standing jobs with more exuberance. All the dish-washing, vegetable preparing, stir-frying, can be done while you ride a horse, or rock your pelvis, or do the hula. Dance as you turn from sink to stove. Waltz your way to the cupboard. When you reach for something on the shelf, use your whole body and really stretch yourself. Music is a help to dance your way through boring jobs.

If you still do ironing, or work in a laboratory or darkroom sitting on a high stool, try to put at least one foot on a rung that will bring your knee above your hips. This will prevent the muscles in the small of your back from becoming tight and painful. And don't sit in one position for hours; move off and on the stool as often as you can.

This brings us to the interesting question of how long should we exercise. I remember a pupil long ago who was pregnant and had a backache. I showed her how to lie on the floor with her feet and legs up on a couch, pillows under her knees, so they were precisely the correct height and her back was hugging the floor. When I saw her the following week, she said that that position did not help her at all, in fact it made her feel worse. I was puzzled until I asked her how long she had remained in that position.

"I stayed there for an hour and a half," she said. "When I got up I could hardly move." Good grief! Why would anyone do that?

She felt, as many people do, that if something is good for you, you should do it till it hurts. Which is, of course, exactly the opposite of what we should do. We need to be kind and loving to ourselves. We need to pay attention to what our body is saying. Of course, the body cannot talk, but it is constantly sending us messages. They are not always loud and strong, so we need to be receptive to them, by quieting our internal dialogue and allowing the messages of strain or discomfort or pleasure to come through.

A new position should be held for only a few minutes, a new movement should be done only once or twice. Your muscles learn more slowly than your brain, so be kind to them, give them time to catch up.

As we get older, we tend to bend over more and more until we have developed a hump on the back, *kyphosis*. The polite name is dowager's hump.

I find that when I am in the kitchen I bend over more than I need to. I catch myself twisted like a pretzel while I cut up an onion or peel a garlic. I tell myself it is because of the darned bifocal glasses. And in a sense it is. You can't just glance down as you did before bifocals, you have to bend over to see properly.

I do have alternatives to bending. I can pick up the garlic clove and bring it nearer to my face as I peel it, and I don't need to see too well to chop things. A good cleaver and a good chopping board are all that is necessary, but it would help to have a work table near the height of my elbow, rather than twelve inches lower.

I can polish the silver by picking it up and looking at it. I can examine the vegetables by picking them up instead of sorting them down there in the sink. And when I really need to see what is cooking on the stove, I can bend my knees and Ride a Horse to get closer to the pot. And, occasionally, I can bend over to examine something closely by bending at the hips while my knees are bent. This keeps the back flat between the shoulder blades.

We all age in different ways and at different rates of speed. The stooped posture is not a sign of aging, it is a sign of disease or of habitual stooping. The trick is to be aware of your body and give it what it needs.

Here is another goodie to help you. Clasp your hands together and raise your arms directly above your head, being sure you keep your arms behind your ears. Stretch a little bit and feel the pull in the muscles of your upper back. This stretch will help to avoid the dowager's hump and is also marvelous to relieve the tightness that comes from sitting at the typewriter or sewing machine for too long a time.

Because of solid furniture like sinks and cupboards, the kitchen is a splendid place to hang on to something solid and swing your legs, first to the right and then to the left. I don't swing as long as I used to, nor does my leg go so high, but it feels good.

I remember going to a conference about arthritis, conducted by the physical therapists at a certain hospital. A young doctor wanted to speak, but as he had not been invited, the program went on and on, ignoring him.

When the meeting finally adjourned, he jumped onto the podium and said, "If everyone who sits for more than an hour at a time would raise his or her feet and legs parallel every hour on the hour, I guarantee that none of those people would end in a wheelchair because of arthritis." He gave no statistics nor proof, but I follow his advice, chiefly because my knees get tired when I sit too long.

Go through the chapter for Sitters once again. Read aloud the movements you like especially well. Do them while you say them aloud. It will take a few days until you find what really feels good to you. Again, you must be the judge of exactly what you do and how you do it. When you say them aloud, you will begin to make them part of yourself.

All of the sitting movements can be used on airplanes and buses, in offices and in your own home, so find the way to make them part of you.

Now I want to talk about what I consider the most important part of the book, the ideas contained in the chapter on Loosening.

Make sure, whether you are standing, sitting, or walking, that you are using only the muscles you need for that activity. This means paying complete attention to whatever it is that you are doing. Remember the work of Dr. Edmund Jacobson: when we think of an activity, the muscles we would use to perform that activity will tighten. The tightening will be imperceptible to you, but your body will know.

How do we remember to keep loose? It is probably the most difficult of all the remembering. When your back is hurting it's easy to remember, "I'll help my aching back by stretching it," but most of the time we are not even aware of tension when we have it. This is a whole new way of thinking—paying attention to our body's situation. Here is a check list.

1.   If you are sitting, are the muscles of the buttocks, lower back and thighs loose, or are you sitting on the edge of your chair ready to gallop.

Two heart specialists discovered, from the upholsterer who was in charge of the furniture of their hospital, that their patients sat only on the edge of the chairs. The fronts of the chairs had to be re-upholstered more often than in any other office in the hospital. This helped the doctors to work out their famous classification of A and B types of people. Among other things, A types tend to sit on the edges of their chairs; more A types than B types have heart problems. So sit loose. Pay attention to the here and now. When you are sitting, just sit.

2.   If you are standing, what about your buttocks and lower back? Are they loose, so that your back can be straight, not arched or swayed?

The arched back with tight buttocks and tight lower spine is the stance of a fighter. You don't stand loosely if you are going to take a swat at someone. It was also the stance of women a hundred years ago, or so it seems from pictures of ladies of fashion of that time. Your stance communicates to others your feelings and your openness to friendship.

3.   What about your hands? Are they loose or are they clenched into fists—like the fighter stance referred to above?

4.   What about your shoulders? Is one shoulder raised higher than the other? Do you have a chip on your shoulder? Do you feel defensive toward others? Are your shoulders hunched up around your ears like a turtle?

A former pupil once said that she liked them up, because, for some reason, the position gave her the illusion that she was invisible. Then she discovered that when she let her shoulders be loose and allowed her neck to be free and long, she not only felt like a queen but her children and her husband treated her with more respect.

When you drive a car, are your shoulders loose or are you pushing against the steering wheel as though it was your energy making the car go? The motor propels the car forward, you just have to steer. You won't be so tired if your shoulders are loose.

5.   What about your jaw? Are your teeth clenched? Is your jaw pushed forward? Do you grind your teeth in your sleep?

This is a terribly expensive habit; dentists get rich because of it. Whenever you think of it, wag your jaw and yawn. Before you go to sleep at night, tell yourself, out loud, that your jaw is loose, your teeth are parted, you are relaxed.

A pregnant pupil, years ago, had the clenched-teeth habit. She learned that when she clenched her jaw, this acted as a signal to the rest of her body to tighten up. She decided that when she went into labor she would let her jaw hang open, even though it made her look like an idiot. When she was in the hospital concentrating on being loose and letting her jaw hang open while she experienced contractions as sensations, not as pain, two nurses stopped by her open door. One said to the other, "Isn't that disgusting, coming to the hospital drunk?" I am proud to say that my pupil giggled to herself and did not take the trouble to correct the nurses. She was too loose to bother.

6.   And now—what about your tongue? Loosening the tongue and stopping the inner dialogue is truly rewarding, for then, as Wuji says, "you can listen to your inner standing."[2] Even if we can keep our concentration for only a few seconds at a time, it is worth it.

When we have lost something, or have been confronted by an insurmountable problem, if before panic sets in, we concentrate for a few minutes on loosening the tongue, thinking no thoughts, we often will be led to the lost object or remember where we left it, or we will know how to cope with the problem. This is hard to do. Sometimes we need a good friend to remind us.

Moreover, being able to stop talking to ourselves is invaluable to both hearing and seeing. Our relationships with people will improve, our perception of nature will be enhanced, as well as our own self-knowledge.

7.   And how are you doing with your Complete Muscular Relaxation? I hope you practice it. It has been a life saver for me and, I expect, for many people.

It may sound strange, but in order to practice complete relaxation, I think you need to say it aloud. Our muscles respond to command, especially to a voice. The idea of this exercise is NOT to go to sleep, nor to drift off to never-never land, nor to have a lovely imaginative trip. Rather, the idea is to think our way *into* our muscles, to concentrate so hard that we actually feel our feet and legs loosening, actually feel the muscles and tendons of our backs becoming soft and loose, our fingers tingling and the muscles of our foreheads, and around our eyes, letting go. We become aware of every part of our bodies.

You will need to concentrate very hard, but with the sound of your voice saying, "Let go, be loose, be loose," you will condition your muscles to doing this. It will take awhile. Do not be discouraged. After all, you have spent a whole lifetime "pulling yourself together." We are opening a door that will give us a new way to perceive the world.

Notes

CHAPTER ONE

1. Edmund Jacobson, *Progressive Relaxation*, 2nd edition (Chicago: University of Chicago Press, 1938), pp. 40-74.
2. Tarthang Tulka Rinpoche, seminar in February 1974. For further information write to Nyingma Institute, 1815 Highland Place, Berkeley, California 94709.
3. Winifred Lucas, author, teacher, lecturer, from a seminar given by the Extension Division of the University of California in Santa Cruz. Seminar was entitled "Visualization: New Directions in Body Mind." December 1979.
4. George Leonard, author and teacher of a class in Energy Awareness in Mill Valley, California. Although I had experienced unfocused eyes long ago, his name, "soft eyes" delighted me.
5. Alan Watts' remarks on KPFA radio, California during 1950-1951.

6. Fritjof Capra, *The Tao of Physics* (Berkeley, California: Shambhala Publications, Inc., 1975), p. 241.

CHAPTER FOUR

1. Jacobson, pp. 332-342.

CHAPTER FIVE

1. Mary Sue Fitzgerald, "Renewal," *Six by Six is Thirty-six,* (Lagunitas, California: The Owl Press, 1976), pp. 25-26.
2. Lewis Thomas, *The Lives of a Cell,* (New York: The Viking Press, 1974), p. 3-5.
3. Ibid. p. 4.
4. Ibid.
5. Capra, p. 11.

CHAPTER SIX

1. Joel Kirsch, psychologist in Mill Valley, California, and co-author with George Leonard of a forth-coming book, *Energy Awareness in Human Potential.*
2. Betty Grayson and Morris I. Stein, "Attracting Assault: Victims' Nonverbal Clues," *The Journal of Communication,* Winter, 1981, P.O. Box 13358, Philadelphia, pp. 68–75.
3. Ibid, p. 74.
4. Wuji, a ninety-one year old mystic born in Denmark, lived for forty-five years in India. He is known as Shunyata. His words are being collected by friends in the hope that some day they will be published. Wuji now lives in Mill Valley, California.
5. Ibid.

CHAPTER SEVEN

1. Dorothy A. Hughes, *Popular Therapeutic Activity: A Neighborhood Support Group,* p. 1. She is Executive Director of the Mental Health Association of Marin County, California. The article was prepared in January, 1981, but is not yet published.
2. Ibid. pp. 4–10.

CHAPTER EIGHT

1. Arthur C. Guyton, M.D., *Basic Human Physiology, Normal Functions and Mechanics of Disease,* 2nd ed. (Philadelphia, London, Toronto: W. B. Saunders Co., 1977), pp. 202–203.
2. Wuji.

Other titles from Seabury:

Jean Hersey
The Touch of the Earth
"*The Touch of the Earth* shares one very special year in the lives of Jean and Bob Hersey, as they savored their almost idyllic life in mountainous Tryon, North Carolina....[the book] is really about the quality of life and the threads that make life rich and meaningful."
2306-7   —*Christian Herald Family Bookshelf*

Mary Lewis Coakley
Not Alone: For the Lord Is Nigh
"The author has done a magnificent job of communicating her feelings and emotions through the printed word. *Not Alone* is a book which I share with my friends."
2324-5   —*The Review of Books and Religion*

Alice Benjamin and Harriet Corrigan
Cooking with Conscience: A Book for People Concerned about World Hunger
Fifty-two healthful meals based on vegetable protein, milk, and eggs. 0902-1

Marny Smith
Gardening with Conscience: The Organic-Intensive Method
Explains how anyone with earth, sun, water, and an interest in gardening can grow enough vegetables to feed a family by using organic methods known for thousands of years. 2325-3